First stage trauma treatment:

A guide for
mental health professionals
working with women

Written by: Dr. Lori Haskell

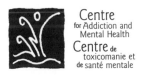

Centre
for Addiction and
Mental Health
Centre de
toxicomanie et
de santé mentale

A Pan American Health Organization /
World Health Organization Collaborating Centre

National Library of Canada Cataloguing in Publication
Haskell, Lori, date
   First stage trauma treatment : a guide for mental health professionals working
with women / Lori Haskell.
   (Women and trauma series)
   Includes bibliographical references.
   ISBN 0-88868-414-2
   1. Post-traumatic stress disorder—Treatment. 2. Women—Mental health.
I. Centre for Addiction and Mental Health. II. Title. II. Series.
RC552.P67H37 2003   616.85'21   C2003-900007-9

ISBN 0-88868-414-2
PG113
Printed in Canada

For information on other Centre for Addiction and Mental Health
resource materials or to place an order, please contact:
Marketing and Sales Services
Centre for Addiction and Mental Health
33 Russell Street
Toronto, ON M5S 2S1
Canada
Tel.: 1-800-661-1111 or 416-595-6059 in Toronto
E-mail: marketing@camh.net
Web site: www.camh.net

Acknowledgment

I would like to express my deep gratitude to Melanie Randall not only for her painstaking and patient editing of this lengthy manuscript, but also for her encouragement, support and unwavering belief in my ability to write this book.

I would also like to thank Barbara Dorian, Kathy Dance and Ursula Kasperowski for their repeated reviewing of this guidebook and for their thoughtful and informed suggestions.

Finally, I would like to thank Margo Kennedy, Joanne Bacon and Myra Lefkowitz for their inspiration and their dedication to working to end violence against women and children.

Lori Haskell, psychologist

Project Team

Author: Lori Haskell, EdD, C.Psych.
Project Manager: Julia Greenbaum, BSC, MA

We acknowledge the following Centre for Addiction and Mental Health staff whose involvement with this project was instrumental in its evolution:

Barbara Dorian, MD, FRCPC
Ursula Kasperowski, EdD, C.Psych.

Additional Contributors

We also acknowledge the following Centre for Addiction and Mental Health staff whose input into the planning of earlier versions of this project assisted in its development:

Marissa Amaroso, MSW, RSW
Barbara Everett, MSW, PHD
Marilyn Herie, PHD, RSW
Teresa Naseba Marsh, MA, RN, OCN
Rhonda Mauricette, BSC, MA
Ellie Munn, BSW
Cheryl Rolin-Gilman, RN, MN, CPMHN(C)
Melanie Trossman, MSW, RSW

Gratitude is extended to the following reviewers for providing helpful feedback on earlier versions of this book:

Giovanna Buda
Rideauwood Addictions and Family Services
Ottawa, Ontario

Dr. Kathryn Dance
Student Development Centre
The University of Western Ontario
London, Ontario

Joan Hurley
Women Abuse Team
Jewish Family & Child Services
Toronto, Ontario

Anu Lala
Women's Health in Women's Hands
Toronto, Ontario

Susan Macphail
London East Community Mental Health Services
London, Ontario

Cherie Miller
The Jean Tweed Centre
Toronto, Ontario

Jan Richardson
University of Western Ontario
London, Ontario

Gosia Wasniewski
Toronto Western Hospital
Toronto, Ontario

Dr. Diane K. Whitney
London Health Science Centre
London, Ontario

CAMH Production Team
Development: Julia Greenbaum
Editorial: Diana Ballon, Sue McCluskey
Design: Mara Korkola
Print production: Christine Harris
Marketing: Bernard King, Rosalicia Rondon

Contents

Introduction

WHY THIS GUIDEBOOK?

Many women seeking treatment for depression, suicidal feelings, substance use problems, difficult or abusive relationships and self-inflicted harm may actually be experiencing complex post-traumatic stress responses. These responses most often result from a history of chronic abuse or neglect in childhood. While post-traumatic stress disorder (PTSD) has been recognized for some time, complex PTSD is a recently recognized diagnostic category. It is a category that better captures the range of adaptations and effects of trauma resulting from early and/or chronic child abuse — abuse that is most often perpetrated in a larger context of neglect and deprivation.

Many mental health professionals are aware that their clients have histories of abuse and neglect that have resulted in post-traumatic stress. However, they can underestimate the degree to which the trauma has been pathogenic, or the origin of their responses (or symptoms). Mental health professionals sometimes focus in a fragmented way on different symptoms (e.g., depression, inability to maintain close, intimate relationships and panic attacks), not realizing that the client's apparently chaotic presentation reflects underlying complex post-traumatic stress.

An increased understanding of the pervasive role of psychological trauma in the lives of clients with histories of abuse and neglect will lead to more effective and appropriate treatment approaches.

SIMPLE AND COMPLEX POST-TRAUMATIC STRESS — WHAT IS THE DIFFERENCE?

Because simple and complex post-traumatic stress disorders are two distinct diagnostic and descriptive categories, it is important to understand the differences between them. (These differences are elaborated more fully in subsequent sections of the guidebook.)

Simple post-traumatic stress

In brief, **simple post-traumatic stress disorder** (simple PTSD) typically results from a one-time terrible event, such as a rape or a serious car accident.

1

To be given a clinical diagnosis of PTSD, certain criteria must be met. These include:

A. experiencing an event in which the life, physical safety or physical integrity of the client was threatened or actually harmed, resulting in feelings of intense fear, helplessness or horror

B. continuing to re-experience the **traumatic event** after it is over

C. seeking to avoid reminders of the event

D. exhibiting signs of persistent arousal

(American Psychiatric Association, 1994)

Complex post-traumatic stress

By contrast, women with **complex post-traumatic stress disorder** (complex PTSD) have often experienced chronic and repeated abuse in intimate relationships throughout their lives. Women with these experiences often mistrust others and, understandably, tend not to believe in the existence of safety. Complex PTSD includes the impairment or destruction of the capacity to trust and the loss of faith that safety is possible. Usually, the client's feelings of trust, which existed before the abuse, are replaced by an active and pervasive expectation of harm, exploitation and further betrayal. As a result, the body and mind are continuously mobilized, anticipating the need for self-protection.

Complex PTSD is multi-dimensional and pervasive because it is often the result of ongoing damaging and neglectful experiences, and is frequently compounded by a childhood that lacked consistent, predictable and attuned parenting. Because of this, the effects of complex PTSD are typically more far-reaching than simple PTSD and affect six dimensions of psychological functioning (detailed in the following sections of the guidebook). Simple PTSD affects only three dimensions of psychological functioning.

> Note: Individuals who have had severe and frightening experiences as children or as adults can have complex PTSD and not have simple PTSD, but usually they have both (Luxenberg, Spinazzola & van der Kolk, 2001).

GOALS OF THIS GUIDEBOOK

The major goals of this guidebook are to:

- expand and deepen mental health professionals' knowledge of complex post-traumatic stress responses (which include depression, suicidal feelings, substance use problems, difficult or abusive relationships and self-inflicted harm).
- address the common clinical error of uncovering and exploring clients' traumatic experiences before they are equipped to do so. Establishing the foundation to do this later work is an arduous and complex process. Highly skilled clinicians need to help clients develop initial stabilization and containment strategies, using a variety of clinical techniques and approaches.
- present the biological, psychological and social contexts of trauma and its treatment. This includes a gender-sensitive analysis that grasps the significance of women's unequal gender status in society and also takes into account other social inequalities such as those of class, race, ability and sexuality.
- give a greater appreciation and understanding of the multi-dimensional nature of complex post-traumatic stress responses and the complexity of treatment.

Greater awareness of what causes the various mental health difficulties associated with complex post-traumatic stress has resulted in a profound shift in the services and treatment offered to women who have experienced abuse-related trauma.

One consequence of this shift is that phase-oriented trauma treatment is now the standard approach.

> Clinicians agree that treatment for clients who have histories of abuse and neglect should be conducted in a series of distinct therapeutic stages (Courtois, 1999; Chu, 1998).

The concept of stage-oriented treatment is based on extensive clinical experience demonstrating that many survivors of severe childhood abuse require an initial and often lengthy period to develop fundamental skills before they can explore or process their childhood traumatic events.

WHO SHOULD READ THIS GUIDEBOOK?

Most mental health professionals recognize the challenges and difficulties in offering help when a client's problems seem complex and overwhelming — both for the client and for the caregiver. Professionals may feel unsure about how best to intervene. In developing this guidebook, mental health service providers — including emergency nurses, alcohol and drug counsellors, psychologists, psychiatrists and social workers — working in varied settings were surveyed about what kind of information on treatment approaches to trauma would be helpful. Those surveyed expressed a strong interest in learning more about ways to increase their clients' safety and reduce and stabilize responses to trauma in the lives of the women abuse survivors with whom they work.

This guidebook has therefore been written specifically for professionally trained mental health workers who are actively engaged in treating women abuse survivors and for related caregivers who wish to understand more about the lives of the clients they serve. Because this guidebook is written with a multidisciplinary audience in mind, the terms therapist and mental health professional are used interchangeably throughout.

Women experiencing complex post-traumatic stress responses may seek help through any number of services. While the focus of this guidebook is on trained mental health professionals providing first stage trauma treatment, some of the information in this guidebook is relevant for a somewhat broader and more diverse audience. For example, some front-line workers who may deliver supportive services that are not actually psychotherapy may wish to better understand the complex set of trauma responses often manifested in abuse survivors, and they may want to know more about the components of first stage trauma treatment for women. Such knowledge can be useful when making referrals or finding suitable additional resources for women abuse survivors. Selected specialized terminology, appearing in bold type, is defined in the glossary at the end of this book.

OVERVIEW OF THIS GUIDEBOOK

This guidebook provides a conceptual map for understanding women's experiences of trauma, outlines the basic components of first stage trauma treatment, and offers specific tools and concrete strategies to use in beginning this work.

It is conceptualized as a resource for therapists who work with clients who experience simple or complex post-traumatic stress responses.

Part I
Part I begins with a review of the nature of both simple and complex post-traumatic stress. Next, there is a discussion of biological and psychological responses to traumatic experience(s) and the role of the social contexts in which neglect and abuse — particularly violence against women and children — are perpetrated. The combination of biology, psychology and social context gives rise to responses in six areas of psychological functioning for people with complex PTSD. These dimensions are discussed in depth in the sections that follow.

Part II
The sections in Part II clarify and explain a first-phase treatment approach. They also address clinical challenges in trauma therapy and how to diagnose the need for specialized trauma treatment.

Part III
Techniques and strategies needed to effectively conduct this work with trauma clients can be found in Part III. The information about complex trauma responses and the specific skills and interventions offered in this guidebook should help mental health professionals face the clinical challenges inherent in this work with greater ease and, ultimately, greater effectiveness.

A NOTE ABOUT LANGUAGE
It is extremely important that the language used by mental health professionals to describe and identify the issues women are struggling with is accurate, sensitive, respectful and appropriate. It is also crucial to use language that avoids stigmatizing clients with abuse histories or pathologizes their ways of coping. The language should also more accurately and respectfully capture the essence of their experiences.

Using more appropriate language is part of a broader commitment to develop respectful mental health approaches to describe and work with the effects of violence and abuse in women's lives.

Too often, the traditional language and terminology used in the mental health field has been problematic — it has pathologized those who seek and use mental health services. Some key examples are explained below with suggestions for terms that avoid, or at least minimize, this problem.

"Responses" instead of "disorders"

The term post-traumatic stress "disorder" identifies the person experiencing stress from a traumatic event as having an internal psychological "illness." This label implies that there is something wrong with the person, rather than acknowledging that the person is dealing with typical and normal repercussions from having experienced a traumatic life event or events. It is crucial to find language that identifies the psychological effects while avoiding constructing a label or identity that stigmatizes the person experiencing these effects.

Meichenbaum (1994) suggests that to avoid pathologizing the client's condition, the therapist can use the term post-traumatic reactions or "responses" instead of the term post-traumatic stress disorder. This terminology will relieve some clients, particularly if they have previously received multiple psychiatric diagnoses. Other clients may feel that the term "responses" minimizes the extreme nature of their experience. Skilled clinicians will choose language that takes into account their clients' specific preferences and needs.

Wherever possible, instead of using the term "syndrome" or "disorder," this guidebook uses the term "post-traumatic stress responses" (PTSR) to capture the ways in which the effects of trauma are typically experienced. However, the literature in the field and the emerging diagnostic category continues to refer to complex PTSD. This results in some unavoidable inconsistency throughout the text.

"Adaptations" instead of "symptoms"

The term "symptoms" suggests a traditional medical model (or framework) for understanding abuse and the related traumatic effects on women's lives, which does not take into account the context of abuse or adequately grasp its long-term effects. The term "symptoms" is less effective in this regard, and is more appropriate in discussions of diseases. The terms "adaptations," "effects" and/or "responses" better capture the ways in which people cope with abuse and other traumatic events in their lives. These terms will be used whenever possible throughout the text.

Clients/patients

The same concerns surround the best terminology for referring to the women (and men) with whom therapists work in their clinical practices. While the term "patient" is restricted to those seen in professional medical practices, the term "client" (despite its unfortunate commercial connotations) more accurately describes people seen in a range of professional mental health contexts. There has been a move toward describing those making use of mental health services as "consumers." However, the commercial connotations of this term are even starker, making it a less appropriate descriptor.

Survivors/victims

There is also a move to describe those who have experienced childhood sexual abuse as "survivors," instead of victims. While the term "victim" tends to label the person in terms of what has been done to her, the term "survivor" highlights the strengths and resilience she uses in coping with abuse experiences. For this reason, this guidebook uses "survivor" wherever possible, but also refers to "women who have experienced abuse" to reduce the use of labels.

PART I
The Biological, Psychological and Social Contexts of Trauma: A Conceptual Model

Part I of the guidebook offers a conceptual framework through which to understand the prevalence and effects of abuse and violence in women's lives and the ways in which this can manifest in complex post-traumatic stress responses. This framework does not assume a linear relationship between the experiences of abuse and the onset of complex post-traumatic stress responses. Instead, it explains how other significant factors in a woman's life might contribute to the development of these disparate and complex psycho-physiological adaptations.

Part I also discusses the role of gender and its connection to mental health issues in women's lives. As well, it emphasizes the importance of understanding psychological development as it affects trauma. The need for a phase-oriented approach to trauma treatment is stressed, as the first phase is the foundation for any future work.

CHAPTER 1
Abuse and Trauma in Women's Lives: Understanding Gender

Chapter 1 outlines the importance of taking gender and social context into account in understanding the consequences of abuse. This includes understanding the significance of gender inequality and traditional gender socialization:
• in relation to women's mental health
• in the disruption of normal development of self-capacities
• in the experience of post-traumatic stress responses.

CHAPTER 1
Abuse and Trauma in Women's Lives: Understanding Gender

GENDER, TRAUMA AND SOCIAL CONTEXT

Over the past two decades, there has been a growing recognition that significant mental health needs of women have not been adequately recognized or treated (Miller and Sholnick, 2000; Morrow and Chappell, 1999; Kaschak, 1992; Worel and Remer, 1992). Women's mental health needs are often distinct from those of men, indicating the importance of taking gender into account in understanding and responding to the psychological issues of clients.

Women's mental health needs cannot be adequately grasped without understanding the way in which they are linked to and, in many cases, emerge from women's unequal status in society. Gender is not simply an individual difference. Instead, gender is a social status and a status of social inequality, around which an entire set of social assumptions and practices are built. A gender-specific approach to women's mental health, therefore, is necessary both for understanding the mental health issues women most often face and for responding to the unique conditions of women's lives, and the impact of these conditions on women's physical and mental well-being.

Borderline personality disorder and gender

Gender plays a significant role in mental health issues. For example, over 70 per cent of people diagnosed with borderline personality disorder (BPD) are women. Those diagnosed as "borderlines" have been stigmatized as being difficult to work with and treatment-resistant (meaning that they don't respond well to therapeutic interventions).

Key symptoms of borderline that many mental health professionals found so unpalatable were responses of **emotional lability** and profound mistrust and anger expressed in what have been considered to be manipulative and aggressive ways.

There is now much greater awareness that many of the women who have been considered "borderline" are in fact experiencing complex post-traumatic stress responses (McLean, 2001; Briere, 1996). Like complex PTSD, a diagnosis of BPD has been associated with a history of chronic sexual, physical and emotional abuse or neglect in childhood.

The adaptations and responses women typically develop throughout their lives as a result of chronic abuse are shaped and determined by multiple factors. These factors include gender socialization into traditional notions of femininity, sexism, racism, poverty and other social conditions of their lives. The ways in which women are socialized to internalize these experiences and women's greater social powerlessness resulting from gender inequality lead to significant gender differences in women's mental health issues and needs. These differences affect the way in which women's problems are most typically diagnosed within the mental health system.

Despite these differences, there is often little recognition or understanding in the literature on trauma treatment and theory of the actual conditions of many women's lives or of the effects of gender inequality, sexism, female socialization, class and race that influence women's psychological develop-ment. In other words, most trauma theory ignores the role of gender. Yet a failure to take these factors into account leads to a failure not only in under-standing the mental health issues women face, but in providing effective therapeutic interventions.

THE IMPACT OF GENDERED VIOLENCE AND ABUSE IN WOMEN'S LIVES

Experiences of sexual violence and abuse in women's lives instill lessons in, and reinforce, what it means to be female in this society — that is, being rel-atively disempowered and with compromised or non-existent rights to auton-omy and bodily integrity.

The pervasive problem of men's violence in our society, combined with experiences of gender inequality, often reinforce the earlier incidents of threat and danger inherent in the experiences of childhood abuse. Early experiences of sexual violation teach female abuse survivors lessons about betrayal, physical and emotional danger and what it is to be dominated. Even women who have not been sexually abused share the reality of living in a society where there is gender inequality and potential for male sexual and physical violence. Indeed, this is an element of gender inequality itself.

Revictimization

Even after an abuse experience ends, experiences of violation and fear are often present for women throughout their lives, by virtue of living in a society in which violence against women and children is pervasive. The phenomenon of **revictimization** — multiple experiences of sexual violence, as well as the increased vulnerability to further sexual violence, resulting from an early experience of child sexual abuse — is a far greater problem in women's lives than is acknowledged in the literature (Haskell, 1997). In her book *Trauma and Recovery*, Judith Herman (1992) describes coercive control as a major cause of complex post-traumatic stress. She asserts that prolonged, repeated trauma typically occurs in families and in other relationships in which the woman is unable to flee because she is under the control of the perpetrator.

Feeling trapped and powerless is a natural response to being subjected to a perpetrator's control and abuse of power. Many women and children who are abused may be trapped and rendered powerless in physical, economic and psychological ways. The responses to coercive control are numerous, including accepting the perpetrator's worldview that legitimates the abuse; feeling dissociated; losing faith or hope; withdrawing socially or becoming isolated; and feeling self-hatred.

The cause and treatment of complex post-traumatic stress cannot be meaningfully discussed without understanding how socially constructed gender and gender inequality (in which women are seen as having a lesser social value) are entwined with the experience of being traumatized.

Feelings of disempowerment don't end when survivors are free of their childhood abusers. Rather, gender inequality, racism and poverty render many women less powerful, less valued and with fewer resources available to them — as well as at the mercy of others — throughout their lives. These broader structures of social disempowerment typically shape and intensify a woman's reaction to being abused, exacerbating feelings of powerlessness and vulnerability.

Pearlman (2001) argues that contemporary society questions the reality and pervasiveness of childhood sexual abuse, does not acknowledge that people suffer for years after active abuse has ended and does not believe that people often struggle to remember their abuse. She explains that this discounting and disbelief of the reality of sexual abuse are further evidenced by the fact that our society does not want to pay for treatment for abuse survivors. This fact is made visible by the inadequate provision of services for abuse survivors, especially longer-term treatment that is often needed for the resolution of severe abuse.

Pearlman (2001) also claims that these victim-blaming beliefs have widespread cultural influence. Women who have experienced abuse encounter comments that they "should forget about what happened and get on with their lives" and that "people cause their own miseries." The media have responded to the increased attention to abuse by claiming that we are becoming a "society of victims."

Pearlman (2001) argues that misogyny, patriarchy, racism and homophobia must be taken into account therapeutically. In her words, "these are very real, integral aspects of each of our lives, of the context in which our clients were traumatized, and of our psychotherapies with survivors" (p. 209).

UNDERSTANDING ABUSE AND TRAUMA DEVELOPMENTALLY

Part of the conventional approach to working with abuse survivors is to address their feelings of self-blame. Many therapists repeatedly tell abuse survivors that the abuse is not their fault and that they are not responsible for what was done to them. However, they may never provide women with the information they need to develop an alternative explanation of who *is* responsible. To do this, therapists need first to explore with survivors why they think they are responsible for the abuse perpetrated against them as children. It also involves shifting the responsibility for abuse and violence to where it belongs — onto the perpetrators and the society that produces these abusers.

Childhood abuse and the accommodation syndrome

Mental health professionals need to understand children's reactions to child abuse from a developmental perspective in order to reframe clients' narratives of their abuse experiences and correct any self-blaming distortions. The nature and persistence of responses may reflect the ages and developmental stages at which the traumatic event occurred. Incest perpetrated against a child at age four may influence development, experience and functioning in ways that differ significantly from incest perpetrated against a child at age 14.

Therapists also need to be familiar with the adaptive ways that children respond to abuse. An extremely useful conceptual model is the accommodation syndrome (Summit, 1983), which explains children's most typical reactions to dealing with sexual, physical and emotional abuse.

Without requiring survivors to discuss any details of their childhood experiences, the therapist can explain the normal responses that children often have to experiences of abuse and how these coping behaviours lead to subsequent behavioural and psychological problems, including post-traumatic stress. The accommodation syndrome is also helpful in providing a framework to explain the way in which children are developmentally shaped by the experiences of early abuse and neglect. The syndrome captures the complex ways in which the abused child is often made to believe she is complicit in her own abuse.

THE ACCOMMODATION SYNDROME CONSISTS OF FIVE CATEGORIES OF RESPONSE TO AN ABUSE EXPERIENCE (SUMMIT, 1983). THESE INCLUDE:

1. secrecy
2. helplessness
3. entrapment and accommodation
4. delayed, unconvincing disclosure and
5. retraction of the disclosure.

The responses outlined in the accommodation syndrome become entrenched in a child's experience, particularly with intrafamilial violence or when the child has neglectful, unempathic caregivers. The categories describe and explain, from a child's perspective, how the adult's failure to intervene or acknowledge the abuse results in the child dealing with the trauma as an essentially intrapsychic event. As a result, the child internalizes guilt, self-blame, pain and rage.

The accommodation syndrome also explains how the coping behaviours that children typically use to survive the abuse tend to isolate them. In other words, the very ways in which children might cope with the abuse — for example, by acting out — serve to stigmatize them, thereby compounding their difficulties.

Therapists need to understand each child's perspective of her experiences of inescapable, persistent abuse and neglect to be able to clearly explain and help the child understand the development of traumatic adaptations. Many people still believe that a traumatic event has to be an "objectively" life-threatening event to meet the diagnostic criteria for PTSD. Recent changes in the DSM-IV criteria of what constitutes a traumatic experience, however, reflect an increased understanding that what constitutes a traumatic event relates to the individual's own subjective experience of being threatened or overwhelmed and trapped. By definition, all children who are abused are overwhelmed and trapped. These feelings are compounded further if their abuser is also their caregiver, especially a parent or parent figure.

SEXUAL ABUSE IN CHILDHOOD AND THE EFFECTS ON WOMEN'S ADULT SEXUALITY

One of the often-unrecognized long-term effects of sexual abuse and violence in women's lives is the harmful effect on their sexuality. For some women, one of the long-term effects of sexual abuse in childhood is that their adult sexuality — including both sexual feelings and sexual attitudes — was developed in a distorted way, as a direct result of the confusing and abusive sexual violations they experienced.

When abused as children, many little girls are given special attention, privileges and even affection from their abusers, which is part of the process of their sexualization. This is obviously confusing — being sexually abused while also being treated as "special," being favoured, and being rewarded for being sex objects that exist for the gratification of adult male sexual perpetrators. This dynamic sends deeply distorted messages about sexuality and leads to what is often a life-long and conflicted relationship to a woman's own sense of her sexuality. The dynamic is particularly acute when the perpetrator is a girl's own father (or father figure) or another close and trusted family member.

Some women who were sexually abused as girls have learned that sexual behaviour is an extremely effective way to receive male attention. They may have come to believe that they are of value only when they are being treated as the objects of male sexual attention, which is too often intrusive and/or coercive.

Social reinforcement of sexuality

This same kind of lesson is reinforced in a society that obsessively emphasizes that women should be "sexy" and "sexually attractive" to men and should spend a great deal of their time and energy on their bodies and clothes in pursuit of this goal. As a result, some sexual abuse survivors develop a heightened sexualized manner and appearance as a way to feel noticed and valued.

Unfortunately, women who experience sexual abuse in childhood often experience further abuse and exploitation in their adult sexual relationships with men — a phenomenon known as revictimization. To compound the problem, these women abuse survivors are then often blamed for the ongoing victimization they experience because they are labelled as "promiscuous" or sexually inappropriate.

Unfortunately, many people do not understand that this sexual behaviour is an adaptation to early childhood experiences of sexual violation and that this behaviour is then reinforced by our sexist society, in which far too many men have learned to be sexually coercive and/or violent.

Part of the clinical work with abuse survivors entails understanding how **traumatic sexualization** (the distorted shaping of a child's sexuality in developmentally inappropriate ways) and difficulties with sexuality are effects of child sexual abuse.

Clinicians need to understand the larger social context within which abuse occurs: a sexual double standard for men's and women's behaviour, a denial of women's sexual autonomy (rights to bodily integrity) and a socially produced femininity that is geared toward over-valuing male attention and approval. Sensitivity to these issues is a necessary part of the landscape for providing effective therapeutic support to women abuse survivors with post-traumatic stress.

THE LIMITATIONS OF TRADITIONAL PSYCHIATRIC DIAGNOSES IN UNDERSTANDING ABUSE-RELATED POST-TRAUMATIC STRESS

Many traditional psychiatric and psychological categories and approaches are not gender sensitive and do not account for or address the ways in which abuse and trauma factor into women's lives and shape women's mental health issues. Judith Herman (1992), for example, argues that current psychiatric categories are not constructed in a way that adequately reflects the experiences of survivors of extreme trauma.

Multiple diagnoses and pathology

Many trauma survivors who have sought mental health services have been given multiple diagnoses such as bipolar disorder; schizophrenia, paranoid type; and borderline personality disorder. These diagnoses are descriptive labels for "symptoms" and behaviours that emphasize pathology.

Traditional diagnoses like these typically fail to consider the contexts (the traumatic event/s) in which a person may have developed these responses. In other words, many mental health "symptoms" that women exhibit represent their intuitive and automatic attempts to cope with and adapt to traumatic stress, often stemming from prolonged abuse experiences. Traditional psychiatric diagnoses tend to focus on what is "wrong" with the woman, rather than recognize the ways in which she has reacted to and coped with traumatic events in her life.

Until recently, most mental health professionals failed to understand these problems as part of a spectrum of complex, psychological and physical responses to multiple traumas across a lifespan. Instead, these problems were considered to be co-occurring conditions (van der Kolk, 2001). For example, it is not unusual in a traditional psychiatric setting for a woman to be diagnosed with major depression, panic disorder, borderline personality disorder and a chronic pain disorder with medical and psychological features, without any connection being made between her responses, the mental health issues she exhibits and her earlier experiences of abuse and/or neglect.

The consequences of multiple diagnoses

Not understanding the chronic and complex psychological harm done to abuse survivors has serious consequences for the adequacy and effectiveness of therapeutic treatment. Survivors end up getting treated for an array of "symptoms" and problems as they fit into existing diagnostic categories, without their problems being linked to the traumatic events to which they were responding.

The result is not only a fragmented approach to treatment (Herman, 1992, p. 119), but also the potential for inappropriate treatment because the underlying issues of trauma and neglect have not been identified and addressed. Thus, abuse survivors may not be provided adequate symptom relief and may suffer the additional consequence and possible humiliation of being considered "treatment-resistant" or "difficult patients." This kind of labelling compounds the problem and stigmatizes the women whose lives have been harmed by experiences of abuse.

ABUSE, VIOLENCE AND COMPLEX POST-TRAUMATIC STRESS

Many of the women who have experienced violent or traumatic events in their lives clearly suffer severe and devastating effects. However, the developmental, emotional and psychological consequences caused by violence and trauma, especially originating in childhood, are frequently underestimated and misunderstood by mental health professionals. The complexity of responses has not been fully understood, in part, because the acts of childhood physical and sexual abuse are so abhorrent that these events in themselves have often been thought to create most of the long-term effects.

The context of neglect

It is now better understood that child abuse often happens in a context of severe neglect, emotional invalidation and deprivation (Briere, 1996; Chu, 1998). The effects of emotional and physical neglect are now recognized as contributing to the long-term emotional and psychological difficulties many abuse survivors experience. Neglect may mean not having a parent who is attuned to and aware of the child's emotional feelings and needs, not being protected and experiencing repeated loss and separation.

21

The effects of trauma on development

Cognitive, affective and psychosocial development are shaped and affected by a combination of chronic abuse, lack of emotionally connected parenting and/or the deprivation of basic childhood needs such as safety, parental constancy and emotional validation.

Women who grow up with childhoods characterized by abuse and neglect very often struggle with a host of psychological difficulties. They may have a distorted sense of self, trouble forming and maintaining relationships, an inability to regulate their emotional responses (affect dysregulation) and a belief that people are not safe and should not be trusted. They may also develop substance use problems and engage in other forms of self-destructive behaviour.

These trauma-related processes result in inadequately developed **self-capacities**. Self-capacities are the inner abilities that allow people to manage their intrapersonal worlds and maintain a coherent and cohesive sense of self (McCann Pearlman, 1990). The three self-capacities considered especially important to the individual's response to aversive events are identity, boundary and affect regulation (Briere, 1996).

Identity

Identity refers to a stable sense of self and a consistent internal locus of conscious awareness (an ongoing conscious awareness of self). A strong sense of identity allows an individual to face adversity from a secure internal sense of self. Briere (1996) explains that people with a less stable identity may **fragment** when they most need to have an awareness of their own needs, perspective and entitlement.

Boundary

Boundary refers to an individual's awareness of the distinction between self and other (Briere, 1996). People with poorly developed boundaries have difficulty determining what their own needs and perspectives are, and what are those of the other person. This can result in either allowing others to intrude on them, or in their intrusions upon others (Elliott, 1994).

Affect regulation

The third self-capacity is **affect regulation**, which is the ability to experience, tolerate and integrate feelings (Pearlman, 2001).

Abuse survivors with inadequately developed self-capacities rely on **dissociation** or other external ways of dealing with painful internal experiences. Unfortunately, these attempts to deal with overwhelming pain are not effective in the long term. Women often seek out therapy or help when the adaptations begin to lose their effectiveness.

CHAPTER 2
Attachment Theory and Trauma

Chapter 2 describes:

- the normal development of self-capacities
- the role of attachment theory in the development of self-capacities
- the disruptions of attachment in relation to trauma.

CHAPTER 2
Attachment Theory
and Trauma

ATTACHMENT AS THE REGULATOR OF
EMOTIONAL AROUSAL

Attachment theory plays a critical role in explaining that it is through attachment that infants develop affect (emotional) regulation. **Affect dysregulation** describes the tendency to become easily overwhelmed and disorganized by small stressors. It is a central element of complex post-traumatic stress responses.

Secure attachment

Longitudinal research on attachment shows that early significant relationships in childhood promote lifelong emotional well-being, social competence, cognitive functioning and resilience in the face of adversity (Carlson, 1998). Children depend on their parents to help them regulate their emotions. Parents who soothe their children — for example, by stroking, rocking, feeding, talking and singing to them — help children change their internal states from agitated and unhappy to calm and contented. Adults who are primary caretakers of children are known as "attachment figures."

Secure attachment develops when parents or primary caretakers respond sensitively to their child's emotional needs and signals. Emotionally attuned "attachment figures" or parents amplify the child's positive emotional states and, at the same time, help to soothe and contain (or modulate) distressing feelings such as fear, anxiety or sadness (Siegel, 1999). They help children modulate their physiological arousal by providing balance between activities that are soothing and stimulating. In so doing, they regulate normal child play and exploratory activity.

Children instinctively go to a protective adult when they are distressed or afraid. Nurturing parents establish physical contact and comfort by picking up and holding an upset child, using their voice to soothe them, and/or making eye contact.

In essence, the attuned parental relationship allows for the immature and developing infant brain to develop its capacity to process emotion appropriately.

This is not a one-time experience but a critical ongoing phase of infant development. The developing child is able, over time, to internalize the parents' consistent, sensitive and attuned way of relating. Neural networks are established in the child's brain, allowing for the development of a cognitive map. The map helps the child recognize and respond to emotion states (Siegel, 1999; Allen, 1995; Schore, 2001).

A child thus learns emotional (affect) regulation through secure attachment to emotionally attuned parents.

Insecure attachment

Children who are insecurely attached, on the other hand, often develop a pattern of ambivalent or avoidant attachments later in life. This makes these children more vulnerable (at greater risk) when facing difficult or stressful events. Without being able to establish close, warm relationships as children, they typically will not be able to develop adequate social supports or take comfort from others as adults. They often appear aloof or withdrawn as adults. This makes them even more isolated, as others don't understand that such avoidant behaviour is the way they have adapted to their past experiences.

Young children often soothe themselves by sucking their thumb, averting their gaze and, in extreme cases, dissociation. Dissociation allows infants to disconnect from sensory input by entering a trance state (van der Kolk, 1994). However, infants and young children dissociate primarily to compensate for lack of soothing from their parents. This demonstrates the critical role that secure attachment plays in allowing children to develop affect regulation.

INSECURE ATTACHMENT, ISOLATION AND DISCONNECTION

Attachment is the basis for our sense of safety and security in the world (Allen, 1995). The need for comfort and soothing is evident in all our relationships and is especially prominent with young children. However, women who have been abused (as children, by primary caretakers or, as adults, by intimate partners) learn that relationships are a place where they are exploited and victimized. When they are distressed, they don't seek connections with others as solace or a place to feel understood. Instead, many adult abuse survivors retreat into isolation, relying only on their own internal resources.

This, in turn, reinforces their isolation and sense of disconnection. They may attempt to numb themselves with alcohol or other drugs, with other self-harming behaviours or by immersing themselves in their work or other activities. Their coping behaviours are often effective for a long period of time.

EXAMPLE: DISCONNECTION AND ISOLATION

Disconnection and isolation can be seen in the case of a woman who is an abuse survivor, and who has, for several years, maintained a successful, though isolated, career as a writer. The success of her writing has fulfilled many of her emotional needs, but at night, when she's not working, she drinks to numb her anxiety and feelings of loneliness. Eventually, her drinking interferes with her health and her ability to write. She seeks therapy to deal with her drinking, but she lacks the resources to deal with her sense of isolation.

ATTACHMENT AND THE THERAPEUTIC RELATIONSHIP

The functioning of the mind is shaped by experiences throughout life, not just experiences that happen in childhood. Through therapy, adult clients can learn affect regulation even when this skill was not developmentally nurtured throughout childhood.

As mental health professionals, it is extremely important to offer hope to clients. Having a sense of hope is crucial to healing.

So much grief and loss follows from the damage caused by childhood sexual abuse. It is even worse when adult abuse survivors believe that the harm they have suffered is irreversible.

Clients need to know that they can regulate their emotional states and form secure attachments. Just as abuse and the effects of trauma alter survivors' sense of trust and safety in the world, they need to know that new, more positive experiences can teach them that it's possible to take comfort and solace in other people. The therapeutic relationship is an opportunity to see how a different type of relationship can be formed.

CHAPTER 3
Understanding How Complex Post-Traumatic Stress Gets Produced

Chapter 3 offers:
- a broad conceptual overview of the physiology of post-traumatic stress
- a brief overview of the psychobiology of post-traumatic stress.

.

CHAPTER 3
Understanding How Complex Post-Traumatic Stress Gets Produced

Mental health professionals often deal with the human stress response to trauma in their clinical work. Judith Herman (1992) explains the role of traumatic events on human physiology by pointing out that "understanding the role of trauma and post-traumatic stress ... is a critical component of training ourselves to provide adequate therapeutic care to our clients."

THE BIO-PSYCHO-SOCIAL FRAMEWORK

Trauma can change a person's life when it leads to disruptions in attachment, emotion, consciousness, memory, sense of self and relationships with others. Trauma affects not only women's psychological development. It can also affect their physiological development. In recent years, the increased understanding of the neuropsychological effects of trauma has transformed both our knowledge of trauma and our understanding of effective treatment.

Because trauma affects both the mind and the body, it is best understood in a bio-psycho-social framework. In this framework, all responses and symptoms to trauma are understood as adaptive efforts to cope with the stress of trauma. People physiologically, psychologically, behaviourally and socially adapt to traumatic experiences. Obviously, how girls and women cope with trauma is also influenced by the social context in which they live, including gender socialization. Social circumstances that define and shape women's lives also shape the ways they adapt or cope with trauma.

Recent research on post-traumatic stress responses has further documented the complexity of physiological responses to stress (Yehuda, 1998; Schore, 2001). People use exquisitely complex mechanisms to cope with the various stressful circumstances in their environment. However, there is a limit to the amount of stress to which anyone can adapt. Beyond that limit, the same psychobiological mechanisms that function to allow people to adapt may start to be maladaptive.

PHYSIOLOGICAL EFFECTS:
THE "FIGHT-OR-FLIGHT" RESPONSE

Neurophysiological mechanisms help humans adapt to brief stress but can create further problems in response to prolonged trauma. For example, we are wired to run away from a speeding car when crossing in traffic without any lasting physiological changes. But we are not wired to cope with deliberate, protracted or repeated cruelty. Our body responds to danger and threat by alerting the freeze, fight or flight responses. When this is a one-time event, the momentary anxiety is a useful warning signal and stimulates appropriate behaviour. However, when someone has experienced ongoing and severe childhood abuse, this **fight-or-flight** response is likely to be triggered repeatedly with little opportunity to act in a way associated with fleeing or fighting.

What happens if you cannot fight or take flight?

When children are abused by their caretakers while sleeping in their own beds or when women are battered by their intimate male partners, they cannot typically fight, easily flee or take any definitive action to stop or prevent the abuse. Their instinctual survival responses are thwarted or blocked, resulting in inescapable shock. The inescapable nature of the danger and terror is what makes the situation so traumatic. Often, the woman is trapped physically by the perpetrator's body, psychologically by the perpetrator's threats or emotionally by her attachment to the perpetrator. Or the woman may be debilitated, believing that the abuse is her fault. This is a belief that the perpetrator often seeks to instill in the child.

Blocking this fight-or-flight response causes the emotional reactions to be kept alive long after the original trauma is past, resulting in lingering agitation, tension and anxiety. Chronic anxiety, particularly in the context of ongoing victimization and helplessness, is often debilitating and may give rise to complex post-traumatic stress.

Changes in the sympathetic nervous system

When trapped and terrified, the human sympathetic nervous system (SNS) is activated and there is a surge of physiological arousal.

> Physiological changes during SNS activation include increased heart rate, blood pressure, metabolic rate and alertness, sweating, and blood coagulation (useful if one is injured by a predator); and blood flow away from the skin, gut, and kidneys and toward the heart, brain and skeletal muscles (useful for running away from the predator) (Cohen et al., 2002, p. 96).

Trauma is often thought to involve exposure to a life-or-death experience. However, betrayal by someone you depend on for survival (as a child depends on a parent) may also feel life-threatening. Even though abuse in childhood may not have been literally a life-or-death experience, it is often experienced this way.

The emotional arousal at the time of the traumatic event is often so overwhelming that the woman may need to disconnect from her feelings to survive. The terror and disconnection she experiences is not coded as a typical memory, but rather as a series of disconnected emotions, visual perceptions and sensations.

One theory suggests that an increased sensitivity, or reactivity, to stress may be the reason why some people develop post-traumatic stress responses (van der Kolk, 1994a; Cohen et al., 2002). The stress response system becomes maladaptive and the brain continues to prepare the body for fight or flight even though the actual traumatic event has ended. With this increased SNS reactivity, people with post-traumatic stress responses live with hyperarousal and continue to experience anxiety, panic, muscle stiffness, difficulty concentrating and sleep disturbance.

Changes in the brain's limbic system

Information from hearing, sight, touch or smell is transmitted through neural connections to the amygdala, which is part of the brain's limbic system. The amygdala integrates this sensory information for storage and retrieves the information from memory. It attaches **emotional valence** (weight or impact) to the received sensory information and then transmits this information to all other systems involved in the stress responses. When sensory information is perceived to be stressful, the amygdala triggers both physiological and psychological responses (Eichenbaum & Cohen, 2001).

Overwhelming experiences are stored in the amygdala without conscious control and without symbolic or linguistic representation. Van der Kolk (2001) and others propose that post-traumatic stress responses may result from the hyper-responsiveness of the amygdala. The amygdala is directly involved in attaching emotional valence to sensory information and in encoding, storing and retrieving emotional memories. Its overreactivity "might explain the recurrent and intrusive traumatic memories as well as the excessive fear associated with reminders of the traumatic event" (Cohen et al., 2002).

Working closely with the amygdala is a part of the brain involved in extinguishing learned fear responses (the anterior cingulate of the medial prefrontal cortex). This region of the brain is believed to become underreactive in PTSD and fails to extinguish fear responses that are no longer necessary (Cohen et al., 2002).

The maladaptions of the amygdala and the prefrontal cortex are thought to contribute to core post-traumatic stress responses, including increased and intrusive traumatic memories (flashbacks or nightmares) and the extreme fear that is associated with **triggers** from the traumatic event.

The role of chronic anxiety and fear in trauma

Traumatic memories or automatic triggers can turn on a self-perpetuating anxiety circuit in the brain. Research indicates that high levels of emotional arousal interfere with cognitive (intellectual) processing and that having a flashback interferes with the region of the brain (Broca's area) needed to put feelings into words. Extreme arousal of emotions also makes it impossible for the brain to properly assess and organize incoming information. These neurophysiological effects seem to be responsible for trauma memories being stored as fragmented sensory and emotional traces (van der Kolk et al., 2001).

In normal circumstances, people are able to express their experiences verbally and form a coherent narrative about their experiences. They can emotionally process and find meaning in what they have experienced, and can make this meaning understandable to others. As a result, others can respond empathically to what they have gone through.

However, trauma memories are often relived and re-experienced without being remembered. Survivors often have little or no verbal capacity to represent the event or to form a narrative. As a result, they often cannot talk about their experiences and cannot form a coherent story about them. Instead, they end up re-experiencing unprocessed emotions, images, smells or sounds of the trauma for months and even years after. Because these sensory imprints are re-experienced over and over, many abuse survivors often behave as if they were living in the past and do not realize that these feelings or actions are not relevant or in proportion to what is actually happening in the present.

As van der Kolk explains, when people are experiencing flashbacks they are reimmersed in the experience — they are reliving the trauma and lack the capacity to analyse what is going on in the here and now (van der Kolk, 2001).

Conditioned emotional responses and trauma

After being abused and neglected, survivors often make classically conditioned associations between abuse stimuli and negative emotions (Briere, 2002). These responses are not encoded as normal memories but rather as associations between certain stimuli (e.g., an angry facial expression) and a particular response (e.g., fear and paralysis). These are called **conditioned emotional responses**. Conditioned responses are the automatic ways that a person responds to a particular stimulus or similar stimuli.

Emotional arousal (fear or terror) often becomes disconnected from goal-directed action when people are unable to "take flight or fight." In other words, people who experience post-traumatic stress no longer understand arousal as a cue to pay attention to important incoming information (van der Kolk, 1994). Instead, they tend to go immediately from stimulus (fear) to response (fight or flight), often without realizing what it is that makes them feel so upset and without first appraising the situation. People may do this even with relatively minor provocations that don't seem to warrant this strong a response.

The fight or flight response is automatically triggered whenever the person feels emotionally aroused (e.g., anxious, fearful, hurt or rejected) by events or stimuli similar to the original abuse. For example, a woman who experiences post-traumatic stress responses loses the ability to decide whether an experience requires flight (e.g., escaping emotionally — by dissociating) or whether another type of reaction is possible. The woman cannot simply "take time out" and decide on a reaction; she just responds to the familiar stimuli in the way that she has learned from experiences of abuse. These responses may appear to be "out of the blue." Because the conditioning is non-verbal, the survivor may not even understand why she is responding this way.

When people relive some aspect of their traumatic experience and lack the capacity to understand what has happening to them, they are often further traumatized. This is heightened by the fact that trauma sensations are frozen in time. The trauma-related sensations are experienced as if they are happening in the present rather than things remembered from the past.

> Many abuse survivors believe that they will never be free of these sensory intrusions and that they can do nothing to make them stop. A central task of trauma therapy, therefore, is to help people understand that certain emotional or body (somatic) reactions belong to the past.

CHAPTER 4
The Six Dimensions of Complex Post-Traumatic Stress Disorder

Chapter 4 outlines the six dimensions of complex post-traumatic stress responses:
- affect dysregulation
- dissociation and changes in consciousness
- changes in self-perception
- disturbances in relationships
- somatization
- alterations in systems of meaning.

CHAPTER 4
The Six Dimensions of Complex Post-Traumatic Stress Disorder

Because simple PTSD is a model that is based on a single event, it does not capture or encompass the complex and disparate adaptations associated with prolonged and repeated abuse and neglect. Individuals who have experienced abuse and/or neglect by their own family members have a very different clinical picture than individuals who have survived a car accident or a mugging. Trauma resulting from abuse perpetrated within a close relationship has psychological consequences that are outside the parameters of what is classically diagnosed as simple PTSD.

Recent research on complex PTSD (Luxenberg, Spinazzola and van der Kolk, 2001) demonstrates that trauma has its most profound impact when it begins in early childhood or adolescence. The age at which the traumatic event or events occur is significant because it shapes subsequent adaptation patterns and results in profound changes in attachment, sense of self and relationships.

The diagnostic criteria for complex post-traumatic stress disorder
Extensive research has been done on the development of the diagnostic criteria for complex PTSD or disorders of extreme stress not otherwise specified (DESNOS) (Pelcovitz et al., 1997).

In DSM-IV field trials almost half the sample had experienced a major traumatic experience (in the form of abuse) before the age of 11 (van der Kolk, Pelcovitz and Roth, et al., 1994). Trauma that results from interpersonal abuse — especially abuse experienced at an early age — has pervasive effects on personality and social development. Together, the adaptations and alterations in psychological functioning have been conceptualized as complex PTSD or DESNOS.

The construct of complex PTSD consists of six dimensions, each associated with early interpersonal trauma. The combination of these changes constitute complex post-traumatic stress.

The six dimensions of complex PTSD are:
1. affect dysregulation (the inability to manage feelings and impulses)
2. dissociation and changes in consciousness
3. changes in self-perception
4. disturbances in relationships
5. somatization: physical responses to psychological and emotional distress
6. alterations in systems of meaning.

The Six Dimensions and Social Context

In the clinical literature on complex post-traumatic stress, its six dimensions have not been fully theoretically developed. The following discussion of the six dimensions offers a theoretical elaboration of the key characteristics of each dimension. It includes attention to social context and gender, which necessarily provides an enhanced understanding of how the dimensions are developed in the lives of women dealing with chronic abuse and neglect.

1. AFFECT DYSREGULATION

The term affect dysregulation describes the difficulty some individuals have in managing their emotional experiences. This dimension of complex PTSD is considered to be the core after-effect of psychological trauma.

KEY CHARACTERISTICS OF AFFECT DYSREGULATION ARE:
- chronic preoccupation with suicide
- self-injury
- overreaction to minor stresses
- becoming easily emotionally and cognitively overwhelmed
- difficulty calming or soothing oneself
- alcohol and other drug use
- problems with eating
- compulsive sexual activities.

Because affect dysregulation is a central feature of complex post-traumatic stress, it is important to understand its development in chronically abused women.

Affect regulation

Working to develop affect regulation should be a central focus of therapy. This is because unregulated physiological arousal and feelings of being emotionally out of control are extremely distressing problems for abuse survivors. And their ways of coping with these unregulated emotions are often harmful. Effective and specific treatment interventions in this area are described in later sections of this guidebook.

The foundation of self-awareness and **self-regulation** (self-soothing) rests on understanding the nuances and meanings of physical sensations. All emotional states are based on physiological responses, which are understood and identified in a meaningful way. For instance, we have physical sensations that are generated internally (e.g., hunger or the need for sleep) or externally, by experiences between the self and one's environment (e.g., being faced with a fearful situation and, as a result, feeling an unpleasant physiological arousal) (van der Kolk, 2001).

Part of development involves learning to interpret bodily sensations, to attach emotional valence to them and to take appropriate action (van der Kolk, 2001). Children must gradually learn to differentiate the physical sensations associated with fear from those associated with worry. As part of normal psychological development, they must also learn to tolerate and moderate their physiological arousal.

Children who are bullied by siblings often respond by crying so loudly and intensely that they have to pause to take a deep breath. Their faces are flushed with physical exertion and they appear out of control (high physiological arousal). Parents or caretakers then console them and help them by addressing the wrongful act that was done by their siblings. Within a few moments, the out-of-control, crying children are calmed and able to carry on with their activities. This is an example of affection regulation.

Parents or primary caregivers play a critical role in helping to regulate or control children's physiological arousal by being attuned to their child's affect or emotions and by responding to these emotions in a balanced and predictable way. Developmentally, children gradually learn to become less vulnerable to overstimulation and learn to tolerate higher levels of excitement. They also learn to distinguish increasingly differentiated internal states or emotions (van der Kolk, 2001; Schore, 2001).

The impairment of affect regulation

The development of affect regulation is impaired when children are continuously adused and neglected and are not comforted, soothed and validated by a parent or caretaker. Chronically abused children who do not have a secure attachment to a parent or caretaker not only do not learn to regulate their physiological states, but also have even higher states of arousal due to the abuse they have endured.

The combination of being traumatized and not responded to in a caring and reassuring manner results in chronic patterns of **hypoarousal** and **hyperarousal** (under- and over-arousal). When these children become overwhelmed by physiological arousal and their caregivers fail to help them re-regulate themselves, they do not develop the ability to interpret physical sensations and to use these sensations as guides or signals to know how to act on their feelings.

Many abuse survivors suffer from affect dysregulation. They may attempt to adapt to chronically high levels of arousal by using alcohol and other drugs, injuring themselves, developing an eating disorder, clinging to potentially dangerous partners, attempting suicide or being otherwise destructive. Or they may try to avoid the uncomfortable arousal and sensations by becoming depersonalized, "spaced out" or numb — in a state in which they are unable to recognize or explain why they are in distress or even what it is that they are experiencing.

Behavioural adaptations

Behavioural adaptations that women develop to deal with high levels of arousal are extensive and diverse. Often, women who may appear to be high functioning in their work and social lives are actually keeping themselves busy by working extremely long hours, organizing a constantly busy social calendar and enduring maniacal workouts at the gym to disconnect and distract themselves from feeling constantly tense and agitated. Other women may try to reduce their distress by engaging in high-risk activities, such as shoplifting, frequent anonymous sexual encounters and overusing alcohol.

Without the words or language to define their emotional states or physical sensations, trauma survivors cannot overcome the effects of this physical hyperarousal and numbing (van der Kolk, 2002). Knowing what one feels and allowing oneself to experience uncomfortable sensation and emotions is essential in planning how to cope with these emotions.

When traumatized individuals feel out of control and unable to control their distress, they may resort to maladaptive behaviours in an attempt to soothe themselves. When they fluctuate between extremes of under- and over-arousal, it becomes difficult for them to distinguish their current frustrations from their past trauma(s). They are thus prone to react to the present as if the past had returned (van der Kolk, 2001).

It is critical to understand the need for affect regulation because a central therapeutic task of trauma treatment involves helping trauma survivors safely feel and tolerate disturbing sensations. In fact, Bessel van der Kolk argues that:

> teaching terrified people to safely experience their sensation and emotions has not been given sufficient attention in mainstream trauma treatment. With the advent of effective medications, such as the serotonin reuptake blockers, medications have increasingly taken the place of teaching people skills to deal with uncomfortable physical sensations (2001, p. 11).

2. DISSOCIATION AND CHANGES IN CONSCIOUSNESS

Dissociation is an alteration in consciousness characterized by estrangement from the self or one's environment. It is also a defence mechanism to ward off the emotional impact of traumatic events and memories (Cardena, 1994).

KEY CHARACTERISTICS OF CHANGES IN CONSCIOUSNESS ARE:

- amnesia (loss of memory) or **hypermnesia** (heightened recall) for traumatic events
- transient episodes of dissociation (losing conscious awareness of the "here and now"; a feeling of "spacing out")

> - depersonalization (the experience of feeling like an outside observer of one's mental processes or body: e.g., feeling like one is in a dream)
> - derealization (feeling that the external world is altered, unfamiliar or unreal: e.g., people seem unfamiliar or time seems sped up or slowed down)
> - reliving disturbing experiences with intrusive images or thoughts.

Ability to tolerate strong affect

The ability to effectively tolerate and cope with strong emotions (including positive emotions) is a critical developmental achievement, one that is often disrupted for women who are abuse survivors. Many survivors of extreme child abuse and neglect rely on dissociative defences to regulate and control intense emotions. These include:

- depersonalization
- numbing of emotion
- fragmentation
- denial of reality.

These coping mechanisms are defences (a kind of "off switch" for feelings) that survivors use to protect themselves from being overwhelmed with feelings and realizations and from seeing themselves as vulnerable to others in relationships. These behaviours rarely provide the soothing and balance that survivors require. Instead, abuse survivors often end up alternating between extreme dissociation or constriction and extreme hyperarousal, where they feel flooded and overwhelmed by experiencing an excessive emotional response.

Self-Harm

In a study examining the links between child abuse, neglect and self-harming behaviours, van der Kolk et al. (1991) found that the earlier the abuse occurs, the more self-directed aggression there is likely to be. Importantly, he also reported that individuals with the most severe separation and neglect histories were typically also the most self-destructive. Van der Kolk concluded that child abuse first triggers the self-harming behaviour, which is then maintained by a lack of secure attachments throughout childhood. Van der Kolk (1991) also found that women who experienced prolonged separations from their primary caregivers or could not remember feeling special or loved by anyone as children were least able to use interpersonal connections as an alternative to self-harming behaviours.

Dissociation as an imperfect adaptation

To work effectively with women who have been traumatized and to ensure their safety, dissociation needs to be addressed as part of the first stage of trauma treatment. Dissociation is assessed by determining the degree to which a person fragments a traumatic experience and separates it into compartmentalized components. For example, different parts of the experience can be dissociated: a person can feel numbness in the face of extreme danger, or a person can actually forget (dissociating cognitive awareness of events) a traumatic event.

Herman (1992) eloquently explains that survivors of prolonged abuse have the same coping mechanisms as people in captivity. They become "adept practitioners of the art of altered consciousness" (p. 87). Dissociation enables them to cope with an unbearable reality. In fact, childhood abuse survivors can sometimes develop extreme dissociative capacities.

Several researchers have found an association between the severity of childhood abuse and dissociative symptomatology (Putman, 1989; Ross, 1992). Before further discussion of this relationship, it is crucial to emphasize the importance of understanding and addressing dissociation when working with clients who have been severely abused. Clients who dissociate as a means of coping may be forgetful, may appear to be in a trance or "spaced out" during sessions and will often have gaps in memory for significant portions of their lives. A client not remembering what was discussed in the previous session, or not recalling coping skills or safety plans she has learned creates challenges for the therapy (van der Kolk, 2001).

Psychologist Jon Allen (1995) argues that the term dissociation covers broad territory. He explains that dissociation takes many forms — from feeling "spacey," to having amnesia, to shifting between radically different states of mind (p. 74). Dissociation also includes mind-fragmenting capabilities, which allow for isolated divisions of the mind. Dissociation is an extreme defence that survivors use to escape (or inwardly flee) from disturbing or overwhelming stimuli. One woman described her experience of dissociation as similar to the feeling of walking through a snowfall or being surrounded by a soft, semi-transparent blanket.

Dissociation becomes an ongoing adaptation or skill that alters the individual's consciousness by blunting the experience of current sensory reality. It takes place after an internal or external trigger reminds the person of the trauma. For example, a woman smells alcohol on a man's breath. This sensory memory is triggered and creates overwhelming anxiety for the woman who responds by dissociating.

Dissociation acts both as an adaptation and an attempt at self-protection. It is, however, "an imperfect adaptation," (Allen, 1995) as it typically does not keep traumatic material completely out of the individual's consciousness. Many people who dissociate find that they are prone to intrusive memories and flashbacks. Research has also found that dissociating at the time of the trauma can increase the risk of developing post-traumatic stress responses.

The BASK model of dissociation

Dissociation can also create gaps in an individual's memory and lead to what psychiatrist Bennett Braun (1988) describes as the separation of Behaviour, Affect, Sensation and Knowledge. This is what is known as the "BASK" model of dissociation.

For example, a woman who was sexually abused as a child may experience a bodily sensation — an intense vaginal pain — without the knowledge that she was raped. Or some people may have full knowledge of what happened to them but will have no feelings about it.

3. CHANGES IN SELF-PERCEPTION

Abuse survivors' self-concept is shaped by the sense of powerlessness and stigmatization that trauma causes. Psychologists Finkelhor & Browne (1985) postulate that, when present, these dynamics alter a child's cognitive and emotional orientation to the world and distort a child's self-concept.

KEY CHARACTERISTICS OF CHANGES IN SELF-PERCEPTION ARE:
- a sense of powerlessness
- a sense of stigma and of being different from others
- a sense of guilt, shame and self-blame.

These characteristics are distinct, and yet overlapping and mutually reinforcing.

Powerlessness

People who have been abused experience an ongoing sense of powerlessness from having their will and desires ignored and their sense of autonomy and efficacy continually undermined (Finkelhor & Browne, 1986). For many abuse survivors, the helplessness and loss of control were the worst parts of their traumatic experiences. Being subjected to deliberate, protracted abuse erodes survivors' development of personal agency, or belief that they can have any control over their lives.

This sense of powerlessness is further reinforced and maintained when any attempts that an abuse survivor makes to stop the abuse fail. A sense of powerlessness is also present when the woman realizes that she is dependent on the perpetrator and feels trapped in the situation. The psychological consequences of experiencing ongoing disempowerment are anxiety, fear and a lowered sense of efficacy and agency. For some, this may result in the perception of one's self as a victim. For others, it may result in an increased need for control.

Stigma

The sense of stigmatization refers to the negative beliefs (shame, guilt and badness) that many people develop as a result of being abused. The abuser often blames and denigrates the victim for the abuse that he inflicts. At other times, the victim may blame herself for the abuse to keep believing that the abuser (e.g., a father) is loving and not abusive.

Stigmatization is socially learned and communicated to abuse survivors by victim-blaming attitudes in our society. These attitudes are primarily directed at women and take the form of questioning women's and even young girl's supposedly sexually "provocative" behaviour as a way to explain why they were sexually victimized. Women who are physically abused by their husbands are scrutinized and blamed as well. And women who endure prolonged abuse in a relationship with an abusive partner are questioned as to why they did not leave.

A more important question to ask is: what are the barriers in a woman's life, internally and externally, that prevent her from being able to find safety?

Equally important is to move away from questions that blame the victim for the abuse she has suffered (e.g., by asking what she has done). Instead, more fundamental questions need to be posed about why so many men use violence and abuse in their intimate relationships with the women and children they are supposed to love, and what causes this social problem in the first place.

Guilt, shame and self-blame

People typically feel shame about their experience of abuse, especially when they disclose what happened to them, and get reactions of disbelief, discomfort or blame. The psychological consequences of feeling stigmatized are lowered self-esteem, ongoing feelings of shame and guilt, and a sense of marginalization. Abuse survivors often attempt to cope with these feelings by socially isolating themselves. Or they may try to disconnect from their feelings by using alcohol or other drugs or engaging in other self-harming behaviours. Some people who are marginalized get involved in illegal activities.

4. DISTURBANCES IN RELATIONSHIPS

KEY CHARACTERISTICS OF ALTERATIONS IN RELATIONSHIPS ARE:
- an inability to trust
- an experience of revictimization
- the victimizing of others.

The difficulties that many abuse survivors have in relationships is a result of two traumatic factors: betrayal and traumatic sexualization (Finkelhor and Brown, 1985).

Difficulty trusting others

Not being able to trust is one of the most obvious and straightforward reasons why abuse survivors often have difficulties in interpersonal relationships. Disturbances in the ability to trust create an increased vulnerability to revictimization. That is, these individuals are at greater risk of experiencing additional violence and/or abuse.

Most abuse survivors who have experienced ongoing abuse by a primary caretaker or intimate partner understandably have difficulties trusting others and difficulty believing that they can be loved and respected without also being exploited or violated.

> Not easily trusting and being wary and cautious in relationships are self-protective and adaptive responses. Therapeutically, this self-protective stance should be validated and encouraged.

Trusting too easily

Unfortunately, experiences of exploitation and betrayal do not always result in a response of wariness and caution. Most clinical literature fails to emphasize that disturbances in trust can also result in the polar opposite of what we usually consider difficulties in trust issues — that is, a heightened or intensified trust in others.

Studies on rape and incest survivors have found that trust disturbance resulting from trauma is bidirectional (Brothers, 1995). Survivors with diminished trust in others will be suspicious or **hypervigilant**, secretive and withdrawn. However, abuse survivors can also be so trusting that even when another person demonstrates blatant signs of untrustworthiness, the survivor overlooks or denies the signs.

Intensified trust in others is a survival mechanism just as diminished trust is. For many survivors, the need to trust a primary caretaker regardless of betrayal and abuse was necessary to ward off the intense anxiety and feelings of annihilation that would have resulted in admitting that a primary caretaker was capable of such betrayal and abandonment. It was a higher psychological priority to retain the belief that others are loving and trustworthy than it was to not trust and feel the isolation and disconnection from others.

In the psychological development of individuals who have never been abused or traumatized, the criteria for trustworthiness grow more sophisticated and differentiated over the course of development. But, for trauma survivors who have experienced a shattering betrayal, their criteria for trust remain undeveloped or immature. Like other psychological adaptations, the criteria for trust remain frozen or stuck at the developmental level the children were at the age they were abused.

For example, adults who have not experienced abuse and whose criteria for establishing trust has developed normally find that being disappointed by someone they trusted typically leads to their losing trust in that specific person. The diminished trust is not generalized to all people. However, abuse survivors who have experienced repeated betrayals may lose trust or have less trust in all people after one person they trust has disappointed them (Brothers, 1995).

A person who has not been traumatized by abuse can typically evaluate how and in what situations someone can be trusted. But an abuse survivor, relying on immature trust criteria, may often be unable to make these necessary differentiations. As a result, the survivor will experience numerous disappointments and betrayals.

Revictimization

A disturbance in trust can have an even more damaging consequence when it results in experiences of revictimization. Revictimization refers to the phenomenon of having repeated experiences of violence or abuse by different perpetrators.

Rates of revictimization are extremely high for women who were incestuously raped in childhood (Haskell, 1997; Messman and Long, 1996). In fact, research has suggested that 80 per cent of women who were incestuously raped in childhood experienced another sexual assault after the age of 16 (Haskell, 1997). Some women have revictimization experiences while still children and others may have experiences of several sexual assaults by different men in their adult years.

Rarely does the traditional literature address the larger social context in which pervasive violence is perpetrated against women and children by male intimates and acquaintances.

It is highly problematic, however, to represent revictimization as a phenomenon internally and psychologically produced by its victims, as if the perpetrators weren't responsible for the abuse. Yet the increased vulnerability of child sexual abuse survivors to revictimization largely continues to be explained in the traditional literature by examining the psychology of the individual women. Instead of considering the abusers or the abuse itself, women who experience repeated abuse are seen as having a psychological disturbance or difficulty. This suggests that there is an internal problem with the women and it is this internal problem that is responsible for revictimization (Gidycz et al., 1995; Wyatt et al., 1992). The fact that many men are willing to take advantage of "vulnerable" women drops out of view.

The traditional clinical literature also suggests that childhood abuse survivors tend to seek out and/or attract a string of men to dominate and hurt them because they are destined to repeat the patterns of their most painful experiences (van der Kolk, 1989; Mandoki and Burkhart, 1989). The underlying assumption is that the threat of male violence can be transcended by women who have the correct attitude and who have learned to take care of themselves more adequately.

While it is important to understand the ways in which child sexual abuse affects women psychologically, these traditional interpretations of revictimization ultimately end up blaming the women themselves. This diverts our attention from the fact that all women in our society live with the threat and too often the reality of sexual aggression or violence from men (Stanko, 1990).

Women who are survivors of child sexual abuse will often engage in prolonged periods of social isolation and avoid intimate contact as a way of coping with the abuse they have suffered. They may have difficulty believing that they can love and be loved in a relationship that is free of abuse.

Due to earlier adaptations of dissociation or emotional constriction, women who are child sexual abuse survivors often "shut down." They may not pick up on danger signals or attend to their own feelings of unease, hurt or anger or the other person's inappropriate behaviour. This makes them particularly vulnerable in dating or relationship situations where a man is being sexually intrusive and coercive.

This complicated problem of revictimization can thus be attributed to lacking a healthy template for interpersonal interactions, as a direct consequence of being sexually abused. It is also, and more fundamentally, due to the fact that much of the predatory and intrusive male behaviour exhibited in our society has been normalized and made invisible.

---

5. SOMATIZATION

Many women who have been chronically traumatized suffer from persistent physical complaints that often defy medical explanation or intervention (van der Kolk, 2001). This is a complex post-traumatic stress response referred to as **somatization**. Some abuse survivors experience somatization because the trauma has an impact on a biological level that often gets translated into multiple somatic difficulties.

KEY CHARACTERISTICS OF SOMATIZATION ARE:
- chronic and persistent physical complaints that are difficult to diagnose or treat
- headaches
- irritable bowel syndrome
- chronic pain.

The relationship of neurohormones and stress

Herman (1992), Chu (1998) and van der Kolk (2001) explain how the traumatic stress response involves the release of stress-responsive hormones. When abuse is prolonged, survivors attempt to protect themselves by remaining hypervigilant and physiologically aroused. This results in enduring states of anxiety and agitation with very limited opportunity to return to calm or comfort, and overactive sympathetic and parasympathetic nervous systems (van der Kolk, 2001). The overproduction of neurohormones creates general feelings of anxiety and hyperarousal and can cause difficulty sleeping.

Researcher Yehuda (1998) has also documented that people who have been traumatized underproduce cortisol, which acts as an "anti-stress" hormone. Other researchers have found immune system dysfunction in women who experienced chronic sexual abuse in childhood (Wilson et al., 1999).

Changes in physical health

Chronic trauma may "reset" the body's physiologic functioning because of the physical and mental experience of perpetually being on guard for further abuse. Van der Kolk (2001) and Herman (1992) both explain that this may have negative consequences for basic physiological functioning.

Herman (1992) explains that chronic insomnia, startled reactions and general agitation lead to a host of other somatic responses. Some researchers (Felitti et al., 1998) have found that as the number of traumatic experiences increases, physical health decreases. Tension headaches, gastrointestinal disturbances, abdominal, back or pelvic pain and "acid" stomach are common somatic complaints.

Van der Kolk (1996) explains that, "having lost the ability to put words to their traumatic experiences, physical symptoms may provide some chronically traumatized individuals with a symbolic way of communicating their emotional pain (p. 195)." There are some cases where women may not express psychological distress at all, but simply report chronic physical problems, which they may not understand to be potentially connected to their previous, traumatic experiences.

6. ALTERATIONS IN SYSTEMS OF MEANING

Not surprisingly, many women who have been traumatized by repeated or prolonged experiences of betrayal, violation and abuse have difficulty finding meaning or a sense of purpose in life.

It is not uncommon, for example, that abuse survivors no longer hold the spiritual beliefs with which they were raised. This loss of meaning or purpose is the source of despair and loneliness for many abuse survivors.

This aspect of complex post-traumatic stress is something more fully addressed clinically in the third and final stage of trauma treatment.

KEY CHARACTERISTICS OF ALTERATIONS IN SYSTEMS OF MEANING ARE:
- loss of sustaining faith
- loss of hope
- sense of despair.

PART II
Therapeutic Essentials in Trauma Treatment

This section introduces critical clinical challenges and issues involved in providing trauma treatment. It explains that the standard of care for treating trauma is staged and delivered in phases.

While this guidebook deals with the first stage of trauma treatment, it is important to understand why a stage-oriented model is the standard of care for treating psychological trauma. Therapists also need to know how to determine if an abuse survivor requires this first stage of treatment. This next section provides a description and rationale for this treatment model.

CHAPTER 5
Key Clinical Issues in Trauma Treatment

This chapter offers an overview of the key clinical issues in trauma treatment, including:
- why specialized training in trauma work is critical
- clinical challenges in working with complex post-traumatic stress responses
- the need for a phase-oriented approach
- a description of the stages of therapeutic trauma work
- key components of first-phase trauma treatment.

CHAPTER 5
Key Clinical Issues in
Trauma Treatment

WHY SPECIALIZED TRAINING IN TRAUMA
WORK IS CRITICAL

Providing therapeutic treatment to women with complex post-traumatic stress is an extremely challenging endeavour requiring immense skill and knowledge. The preceding chapters outlined a conceptual overview of the contributing psychological, social and physiological dimensions of complex post-traumatic stress.

It should now be evident from the information provided that trauma survivors' lives and relationships have been pervaded by the damage of childhood abuse and neglect.

For many survivors, the following components of complex post-traumatic stress create the most distress for them:
• physiological responses, including heightened arousal
• a tendency to become overwhelmed and disorganized in response to minor stresses (affect dysregulation)
• not trusting or feeling safe around others
• engaging in self-destructive behaviour as a way to adapt to feeling over-whelmed

Mental health professionals may also experience anxiety in dealing with the complex post-traumatic stress responses of their clients. Some of the most significant are addressed below.

CLINICAL CHALLENGES IN WORKING WITH COMPLEX POST-TRAUMATIC STRESS RESPONSES

Bessel van der Kolk (2002) outlines key clinical issues that make providing effective therapy to trauma survivors complicated and challenging. These challenges are outlined below.

1. Speechlessness

Trauma survivors are frequently unable to verbally communicate the essence of what happened to them. Many times, they simply do not know what they feel. Therapists can validate their feelings and explain the context for the trauma responses. But trauma clients will likely still experience disturbing sensations, and will not necessarily be able to understand or interpret their bodily sensations.

2. Teaching clients to mobilize their defences

Most trauma survivors have had their trust violated and are extremely reluctant to make themselves vulnerable to others, especially when it involves issues that make them frightened or ashamed. Many therapists believe that a safe therapeutic relationship will enable trauma survivors to lower their defences and abandon their distrust, allowing them access to painful memories from their past. However, van der Kolk (2002) suggests that therapists should actually encourage trauma clients to actively mobilize their defences, even with the therapist, and become discerning in who they trust.

Trauma survivors require adequate defences to feel safe enough to remain in a therapeutic relationship and learn to manage their trauma responses.

3. Physiological conditioning

Even after abuse survivors remember the traumatic events, understand how they re-enact these events in their daily lives, re-establish trusting interpersonal relationships and experience safety and competence, they are often still vulnerable to reacting physiologically to reminders of the trauma. This makes them feel as if they are back in the past (van der Kolk, 2002, p. 11).

The goal of outlining these clinical challenges is to emphasize the extent to which working with trauma survivors requires specialized training and knowledge. Many of these challenges have been overwhelming to mental health providers, as often they have not fully understood the complexities of their clients' coping mechanisms. Understanding these complexities and having a set of skills to help clients improve their coping mechanisms makes it easier to work through these challenges therapeutically.

PHASE-ORIENTED POST-TRAUMA TREATMENT

Why should post-trauma treatment be phase-oriented?

Only relatively recently have significant works been published on trauma treatment for adult survivors of child abuse (see Resources, p. 187). Expert clinicians now agree that therapists should treat people dealing with complex trauma using a staged or phase-oriented approach (Courtois, 1999; Chu, 1998). The concept of stage-oriented treatment is based on clinical experience demonstrating that many survivors of severe childhood abuse require an initial and often lengthy period to develop and improve fundamental coping skills (Courtois, 1999; Chu, 1998). Only by developing these skills can survivors more fully, safely and systematically explore memories of childhood traumatic events.

With greater understanding of the complexity of post-traumatic stress comes a corresponding awareness of the many challenges that exist in providing effective treatment for survivors of chronic trauma. These challenges revolve around complex differential diagnoses, relational dilemmas and treatment staging.

What is a phased treatment model for complex post-traumatic stress responses?

In phase-oriented trauma treatment, different tasks and therapeutic strategies are associated with the various phases of therapy. There are three distinct phases, though there is necessarily some overlap between them.

THE THREE-PHASE MODEL OF COMPLEX POST-TRAUMATIC STRESS RESPONSES TREATMENT:

Phase 1

The first phase of therapy focuses on helping clients understand and manage their responses and develop safety and coping skills.

Phase 2

The second phase focuses on helping clients modify and process their memories of the traumatic events. It might draw on such specific skills and techniques as prolonged exposure, cognitive processing therapy and eye movement desensitization response (EMDR). Through this second phase, clients thoroughly explore their traumatic experiences and integrate them into a cohesive and meaningful narrative. Clients are able to explore their trauma experiences by desensitizing the intense negative emotions associated with their memories.

Phase 3

The final phase of trauma treatment involves going beyond the actual experiences of trauma to address other life issues, such as relationships, work, family and spiritual and recreational activities.

The focus of this guidebook is on the first phase of trauma treatment. As this phase focuses on educating clients about trauma issues and helping them to develop coping skills, mental health professionals need an extensive array of tools, techniques and strategies. Elements of this first phase often have to be repeated and reinforced throughout the subsequent two phases of treatment. However, many abuse survivors may never develop the capacity to explore or integrate the original, traumatic experiences. For these survivors, the first phase will be the entire focus of their therapy.

Most mental health community therapists, working in diverse service contexts and locations, will not be able to provide and complete this entire stage of treatment. However, they will likely be able to offer different components of stage-one trauma treatment, such as psychoeducation or specific techniques to help clients manage the effects of trauma. Regardless of the extent of treatment being offered, service providers need an overview of what is involved in this stage of trauma treatment and what approaches they can use with clients.

THE CRITICAL "FIRST PHASE" OF TRAUMA TREATMENT

The first stage of trauma treatment is especially critical since it provides the foundation for all future therapeutic work. Much therapy with women who have been traumatized has failed because survivors first seek help when in a state of crisis or extreme distress, when they are not yet able to engage in in-depth psychotherapy. As a result, they have not developed fundamental coping skills needed to deal with the psychological effects of trauma. Nor have they the skills to delve into and explore past traumatic events. Treatment provided in hospital and outpatient programs most often needs to focus entirely on this initial stage of treatment to help women who come to them in crisis.

This carefully paced and phased treatment model for trauma survivors should initially focus on creating a collaborative therapeutic relationship and helping survivors develop better coping skills. It should also involve helping trauma survivors recognize that their difficulties do not stem from their own personal deficits. Rather, they need to realize that their difficulties stem from the adaptations they were required to make to survive in a social context of gender inequality and pervasive violence against women.

Key components of first-phase trauma treatment
In the first stage or phase of this approach, the treatment is dedicated to reducing and stabilizing clients' responses to improve the quality of their everyday life. This is often the most complex and lengthiest stage of the therapeutic work.

The essential components of first-phase trauma treatment
Stage one of a phased trauma therapy model includes the following essential components:
- establishing a **therapeutic alliance**
- promoting client safety
- addressing the client's immediate needs
- **normalizing** and validating the client's experiences
- educating the client about post-traumatic stress and treatment
- using a gender-sensitive approach so that the damaging ways that traditional gender socialization and gender inequality affect women's lives are recognized in therapy
- nurturing hope and emphasizing client's strengths
- collaboratively generating treatment goals
- teaching coping skills and managing target adaptations of post-traumatic stress responses (intrusive ideation, hyperarousal, avoidance, dissociation)

The first phase of trauma treatment is organized around a series of fundamental goals. These goals aim to empower clients by increasing their knowledge of trauma and its effects and expanding their coping skills to deal with their responses.

Key goals for helping women in first-phase trauma treatment
Key goals that underlie effective first-phase treatment approaches to complex post-traumatic stress responses include:
- increasing clients' sense of control over their lives, by familiarizing them with post-traumatic stress responses and the reasons for those adaptations (see Chapter 8, The Importance of Carrying Out Psychoeducation with Clients; Chapter 9, Explaining Simple Post-Traumatic Stress Responses to Clients; and Chapter 10, Explaining Complex Post-Traumatic Stress Responses to Clients)
- helping clients learn coping skills (see Chapter 11, Working Toward Change: Therapeutic Techniques to Help Clients Manage Their Trauma Responses; and Chapter 12, Strategies and Tools for Managing Complex Post-Traumatic Stress Responses). Some clients will need to tend to neglected medical problems and learn the basics of self-care; for example, proper eating and sleeping habits.
- helping women distinguish between the situations in their lives over which they can have increased control and the societal attitudes, conditioning and circumstances that are part of broader social problems and inequalities.
- helping women recognize that their lives are profoundly shaped by the contexts within which they live. This includes an understanding that prejudice based on race, class, ethnicity, sexual identity, age and able-bodiness can contribute to, or is the basis of, the difficulties women experience.
- increasing clients' sense of safety in their work, home and living environments by helping them to identify areas of potential danger or victimization and take active steps to protect themselves.
- helping clients identify their own responses to trauma and reframe them in a less blaming way.
- helping clients see how their current life struggles have been affected by the trauma and its after-effects.
- supporting clients as they attempt to form meaningful goals and connections with other people (adapted from Matsakis, 1994).

During first stage trauma treatment, the above issues should be the focus of therapy, rather than the traumatic events or memories. *Therapy should not be exploratory.*

Therapists need to keep in mind that abuse survivors do not have the tools they need at this stage to tolerate trauma-focused work. Exploring their traumatic experience before they are prepared can worsen trauma responses and escalate self-harming behaviours, suicide attempts, premature termination of therapy and retraumatization (Herman, 1992; Chu, 1998).

CHAPTER 6
Diagnosing and Identifying the Need for Trauma Treatment

This chapter offers mental health professionals:
- information on diagnosing and identifying the need for trauma treatment
- guidance in determining if clients need more help stabilizing and controlling their trauma responses.

CHAPTER 6
Diagnosing and Identifying the Need for Trauma Treatment

As simple and complex post-traumatic stress responses are different, it is important to compare their clinical definitions. It is also helpful to determine what aspects of complex and simple post-traumatic stress responses clients have, so as to tailor treatment approaches to their specific and individual requirements. Note that trauma clients will not necessarily have every dimension of complex post-traumatic stress, nor will they necessarily meet all the criteria for simple post-traumatic stress.

CRITERIA FOR SIMPLE POST-TRAUMATIC STRESS DISORDER

To meet diagnostic criteria for simple post-traumatic stress disorder, an individual must meet criterion A and the designated responses under criteria B, C and D in the DSM-IV (American Psychiatric Association, 1994). Clients often do not fully meet all the criteria but still have partial PTSD.

Criterion A

Post-traumatic stress is the result of exposure to a traumatic or extremely emotionally and psychologically distressing event (or events). The person must have experienced intense fear, helplessness or horror in response to the event(s).

Traumatic experiences have traditionally been defined as those perceived to be life-threatening. However, many women who experience post-traumatic stress do not believe that their experiences were actually life-threatening. The traditional definition also does not capture the experiences of countless women who survived not only past or present physical and sexual abuse, but also childhood neglect and emotional abuse. Following is a more complete definition: A traumatic experience is an event that continues to exert negative effects on thinking (cognition), feelings (affects) and behaviour long after the event is in the past.

People react to traumatic experiences in vastly different ways. Some of the responses are obvious, such as intrusive memories or flashbacks. Other responses, such as feeling numb and empty, are subtle and difficult to recognize.

While the outward display of post-traumatic stress varies widely, three categories, or "clusters," of responses are associated with simple post-traumatic stress:

Criterion B

A person must exhibit at least one of the following responses:
- reliving the event after it is over through recurring nightmares, flashbacks or other intrusive thoughts or images that "pop" into one's head at any time
- experiencing extreme emotional and physiological distress, such as uncontrollable shaking or panic when faced with reminders of the event.

Criterion C

A person must exhibit three or more of the following responses:
- avoiding reminders of the event, including places, people, thoughts or other activities associated with the trauma
- having less interest in friends, family and everyday activities
- being emotionally numb
- having feelings of detachment.

Criterion D

A person must exhibit two or more of the following responses:
- being on guard at all times
- being hyperaroused at all times, including irritable or suddenly angry
- having difficulty sleeping
- not being able to concentrate
- being easily startled
- constantly scanning the environment for (potential) danger.

CRITERIA FOR COMPLEX POST-TRAUMATIC STRESS DISORDER

The diagnostic construct of complex PTSD or DESNOS is not currently recognized in the DSM-IV as a freestanding diagnosis, but is instead presented as associated features of PTSD. Complex PTSD is expected to be included in the next edition of the diagnostic guidebook, the DSM-V. However, it is unclear if it will be given the name complex PTSD or DESNOS. Currently, both terms are referred to interchangeably in the clinical literature in this area.

Simple post-traumatic stress consists of changes to three areas of functioning, while complex post-traumatic stress consists of changes to six domains of functioning. The diagnostic criteria for determining the presence of complex post-traumatic stress entails that a number of specific changes (outlined below) are present in each of the six domains of functioning.

DIAGNOSTIC CRITERIA FOR COMPLEX POST-TRAUMATIC STRESS RESPONSES

(I) Alteration in Regulation of Affect and Impulses
(A and one of B to F required)
A. affect regulation
B. modulation of anger
C. self-destructive behaviour
D. suicidal preoccupation
E. difficulty modulating sexual involvement
F. excessive risk-taking

(II) Alterations in Attention or Consciousness
(A or B required)
A. amnesia
B. transient dissociative episodes and depersonalization

(III) Alterations in Self-Perception
(Two of A to F required)
A. ineffectiveness
B. permanent damage
C. guilt and responsibility
D. shame
E. nobody can understand
F. minimizing

(IV) Alterations in Relations with Others
(One of A to C required)
A. inability to trust
B. revictimization
C. victimizing others

(V) Somatization
(Two of A to E required)
A. problems with the digestive system
B. chronic pain
C. cardiopulmonary symptoms
D. conversion symptoms
E. sexual symptoms

(VI) Alterations in Systems of Meaning
(A or B required)
A. despair and hopelessness
B. loss of previously sustaining beliefs

Luxenberg, Spinazzola, van der Kolk. Reprinted with permission from The Hatherleigh Company, Ltd., New York. www.hatherleigh.com, 1-800-367-2550. © 2001

Some therapists may assume that they can only apply a trauma treatment model with clients who have been officially diagnosed with PTSD. However, many experts in the field stress that a history of severe child abuse or neglect is sufficient grounds for using a carefully paced trauma treatment model, even if the client does not have a formal diagnosis of complex PTSD (Courtois, 1999; Saakvitne et al., 2000).

Stage-one or stage-two treatment?

There are two methods for assessing whether an abuse client requires stage-one trauma treatment. While these methods are not measures of the construct of complex post-traumatic stress responses, they are nevertheless useful in capturing the elevated adaptations related to post-traumatic stress. These methods examine response severity and help in determining whether or not a client requires the first stage trauma treatment strategies of stabilization and response management.

i) The first method is the Trauma Symptom Inventory (TSI), developed by Briere (1996), which helps to assess a wide range of psychological impacts of abuse and other traumatic events and helps to monitor the client's progress in therapy.

ii) The second method is a list of clinical indicators, developed by Andrew Leeds (1997), which also helps to determine if an abuse survivor requires the interventions and strategies of stage-one trauma therapy. If a client has a number of these indicators, it means that she needs more help in therapy with stabilization and response management.

INDICATORS OF A NEED TO EXTEND THE CLIENT PREPARATION AND STABILIZATION PHASE:

- Client history includes early neglect, abandonment or inadequate attachment to caregiver(s).
- Client has difficulty accurately naming and describing her feelings.
- Client reports or is observed to be easily flooded with feelings and is not able to identify the trigger(s).
- At times of emotional distress, client is unable to speak and cannot articulate her thoughts.
- Client does not use or know standard self-care methods (structured relaxation, establishing a safe place, soothing imagery or exercise).
- Client's account of recent stressful events is unclear or vague and self-critical.
- Client is clearly dysthymic (has chronic, low-grade depression), but does not complain of feeling depressed and considers this just a normal way to feel.
- Client does not trust her own perceptions or feelings as information for deciding how to set limits, assert needs or cope with others.
- Client lacks adult perspective and culturally relevant models of basic human rights.
- Client lacks the skills to enable her to have access to social and economic support.
- Client uses alcohol and/or other drugs or self-harms as a means to regulate her emotional states.

Leeds (1997). Reprinted with permission.

FORMAL ASSESSMENT OF
COMPLEX POST-TRAUMATIC STRESS

In recent years, two clinical instruments have been developed to assess if an individual has complex post-traumatic stress. These are the "Structured Interview of Disorders of Extreme Stress" (SIDES) (Pelcovitz et al., 1997) and the "Self-Report Inventory for Disorders of Extreme Stress" (SIDES-SR) (Spinazzola et al., 2001). These instruments have been invaluable in providing empirical evidence for the validity of the complex PTSD construct (Blaustien et al., 2000).

Structured interview of disorders of extreme stress

The SIDES method is the only instrument that has been validated as a diagnostic assessment tool for complex post-traumatic stress (Luxenberg, Spinazzola & van der Kolk, 2001). This method uses a 45-item interview that consists of six sub-scales corresponding to the six complex PTSD symptom clusters. The SIDES method was developed to measure current and lifetime presence of complex post-traumatic stress and response severity.

The authors of this instrument (Spinazzola et al., 2001) explain that research on the usefulness of the SIDES method has focused on whether it works as a baseline measure of complex PTSD diagnosis and severity. It is not yet known whether it will be useful as a measure of treatment outcome.

Self-report inventory for disorders of extreme stress

The SIDES-SR method is a self-report test that measures baseline severity of complex post-traumatic stress responses and the extent to which baseline response severity and response change over time. This is the only instrument that provides a continuous measure of current severity for each of the six complex PTSD symptom clusters (Luxenberg et al., 2001).

Mental health professionals may feel confused about how to proceed with treatment when the client has already been given a diagnosis other than PTSD. As trauma experts (Saakvitne et al., 2000) note:

> [T]here is not a single diagnosis that is applicable to all abuse survivor clients; rather, individuals carrying any diagnosis can be survivors. Often survivors carry many diagnoses. Abuse survivors may meet the criteria or diagnoses of substance dependence and abuse, personality disorders (especially borderline personality disorder),

depression, anxiety (including post-traumatic stress disorder), dissociative disorders, and eating disorders, to name a few (p. 7).

Mental health professionals without in-depth and specialized training in trauma treatment and assessment may not recognize or diagnose the effects of trauma appropriately. Some diagnoses given to women clients by professionals not trained in trauma treatment or assessment should be treated with considerable caution. The validity of these diagnoses may require re-examination.

Mental health professionals need to keep in mind that *diagnoses are descriptive and not explanatory*. In other words, psychiatric diagnoses list behaviours and symptoms, but do not explain how or why a person may have developed these symptoms (e.g., as a response to traumatic stress and as a way to cope) (Saakvitne et al., 2000).

While diagnoses provide a label for symptoms and behaviours, unfortunately, these diagnoses often become labels for the person. For instance, it is not uncommon to hear clients referred to as "borderline" or "bipolar." Many trauma experts have made comparisons between women who have complex PTSD and women diagnosed with borderline personality disorder (Herman, 1992). However, borderline personality disorder, like other diagnoses, fails to consider the role of abuse in women's backgrounds. These static and incomplete diagnoses have not helped therapists provide appropriate care for abuse survivors (Saakvitne et al., 2000).

It is not easy to diagnose women who have suffered from repeated abuse in childhood, as some may present with only physical responses or with various difficulties such as chronic insomnia and anxiety or troubled relationships. Unless the therapist consistently asks specific questions about whether the woman has been or is being abused, the connection between her current symptoms and abuse history may be missed. Failure to make this connection means that the therapist will have only a partial understanding of the symptoms and will miss the client's core problem, resulting in a fragmented approach to treatment.

CHAPTER 7
Establishing the
Therapeutic Alliance

This chapter emphasizes the importance of establishing an effective therapeutic relationship with clients, based on the key elements of:
• collaboration
• validation and empathic attunement
• empowering clients to make changes
• respectful engagement / active facilitation.

CHAPTER 7
Establishing the
Therapeutic Alliance

This chapter deals with establishing the effective therapeutic alliance necessary for undertaking first stage trauma treatment.

The therapeutic alliance — the collaborative relationship between the therapist and client — is the foundation of the therapeutic process. It is especially critical given the issues inherent in trauma treatment.

It is also critical to maintain a therapeutic relationship based on respect and collaboration with the client. Clinicians undertaking this work must have adequate and specialized training in trauma treatment.

For example, women who have experienced ongoing childhood abuse and neglect often struggle with issues of interpersonal trust and safety, as well as fear of exploitation or disempowerment. For these survivors, entering a relationship with a therapist and disclosing feelings and reactions related to early traumatic experiences is a courageous act, accompanied by a range of reactions, including shame, anger, fear, anxiety and hope. The therapeutic alliance is a major tool to help the client re-examine and deal with these feelings and work through interpersonal conflict.

IN THEIR RELATIONSHIP WITH CLIENTS, THERAPISTS NEED TO ATTEND TO AND MAINTAIN:

- collaboration
- validation and empathic attunement
- empowering clients to make changes
- respectful engagement / active facilitation.

COLLABORATION

Abuse, violation and neglect disempower the child or adult victim. Ongoing disempowerment and fear of betrayal and exploitation are long-term effects of child abuse and neglect. From the survivor's perspective, most interpersonal relationships seem dangerous and threatening.

Most survivors will enter therapy expecting that their relationship with the therapist, with its inherent power imbalance, will carry with it similar dangers to those that existed in the relationship with the abuser. Providing a therapeutic relationship characterized by mutuality and collaboration is therefore essential to this healing work.

Too much care leads to dependency

Courtois (1999) explains that clients will not learn the necessary relationship skills in therapy characterized by an overly care-taking approach, therapy that does not stress personal responsibility and therapy that is non-collaborative.

Chu (1998) also emphasizes that clients can't be "loved into health." He explains that therapists who rely on these strategies are setting up therapeutic relationships that will encourage regression and over-dependence. This type of parental counter-transference results in some therapists taking extraordinary measures to alter the external environment for their client.

> Too much care-taking from the therapist resonates and triggers abuse survivors' deep longing to be parented. This causes them to regress into dependent behaviour, hoping that finally someone will make things better for them, instead of working to develop the skills to do so for themselves.

EXAMPLE: DEPENDENCY

A client usually sees her primary therapist at least several times a week. If she can't see the primary therapist with that frequency, she sees her family doctor instead for emotional support. When her therapist is not available, the client feels abandoned and despairing.

The common therapeutic problem demonstrated in this example is that of enabling the client to use professional relationships as a primary source of support. Clients who develop supports that are exclusively external are often faced with the ongoing problems of having limited control and access to these supports. Instead, the therapist should encourage and teach the client to develop increased internal resources and self-capacities to instill in the client an increased sense of self-efficacy and control.

Dependency with trauma clients

Some measure of dependency, however, is a necessary component of therapy with trauma survivors. Trauma clients, like anyone, have legitimate needs for secure attachment. Mental health professionals often struggle with the complex challenge of how to appropriately negotiate and meet the dependency needs of chronically traumatized clients. Many therapists believe that if clients become dependent on them, it is a problem in therapy that needs to be remedied. Therapists must understand the extremes of dependency that are part of insecure attachment resulting from trauma and neglect.

A foundation of security

The secure base developed in the therapeutic attachment provides a dramatic shift for many trauma clients. Instead of feeling wary and avoidant of attachments with others because of fear of harm, they come to believe that relationships can be the source of safety and comfort. Therapy may be the first time that trauma clients experience consistent care and responsiveness from another person (i.e., the therapist). Working from this foundation, clients are often better able to develop secure relationships with others in their daily lives.

The need for balance

Therapists need a skilled and sensitive balance to work effectively with a client's dependency. Therapists must be able to withstand and work through a client's maladaptive expression of dependency needs without rejecting the client either by terminating therapy prematurely or by having inflexible boundaries.

On the other hand, therapists who allow too much reliance risk having the client deteriorate because too much reliance can make the client regress and feel insecure. Mental health professionals are expected to understand individual differences in clients' dependency needs — according to the client's ego strengths, internal capacities and characterlogical structure —

and must tailor and titrate their availability and responses accordingly.

An ideal therapeutic stance is of supportive neutrality, that is neither over-indulgent nor over-restrained. This helps to develop a therapeutic relationship with enough safety to anchor treatment and rework issues of past abuse (Courtois, 1999).

The process of negotiating a client's dependency needs requires far greater discussion than what is possible in this resource on first stage treatment. However, an effective means of helping clients understand and navigate the process of being in a therapeutic relationship lies in establishing a clear treatment frame.

Establishing an effective therapeutic stance with trauma survivors

The list below, adapted from the work of James Chu (1998), outlines some essential points necessary for establishing a solid and effective therapeutic relationship between mental health professionals and clients.

ESSENTIAL POINTS FOR THE THERAPEUTIC RELATIONSHIP

- Therapists have a need for separate lives.
- A client's unhealthy or insecure dependency on the therapist is dis-empowering and frightening for the client.
- Clients need to find their own internal mechanisms of self-soothing and containing dysphoric affect.
- It is unrealistic to expect that the therapist can always soothe and reassure. Clients need to develop ways to tolerate psychological pain.
- Therapists who try to gratify a client's demands do so because they recognize the client's limited internal resources, but fail to understand the need to help clients develop internal coping mechanisms.
- Unconditional love is not helpful — adhering to a mutually respectful relationship is.
- Therapists provide containment and affect regulation by providing *predictability* and *consistency* — not by extraordinary or "heroic" therapeutic interventions.

(adapted from Chu, 1998)

Maintaining a collaborative and mutual approach may challenge some therapists, particularly if they are concerned and anxious about a client's well-being, for example, when a client is self-harming. In these situations, therapists may want the client to co-operate with their suggestions and make changes quickly. Therapists may feel angry and frustrated when these changes do not occur. But it is important to remember that, for some survivors, being accommodating or compliant with someone in a position of authority can resonate with their abuse experiences, in which they were expected to co-operate and their behaviour was controlled. As Judith Herman points out, "Therapists need to understand the distinction between helping a woman control her own behaviour, and trying to control her" (Herman, 1992, p. 133).

When to avoid collaboration

Unfortunately there are circumstances — for example, when a client becomes suicidal — in which a therapist may have to take actions that are not collaborative. Experienced therapists have learned to anticipate these situations, as well as to negotiate agreements and develop crisis plans with their clients in advance.

For example, at the point of admission, some hospital trauma programs discuss with clients that they will together outline the way the therapist will unilaterally intervene and/or restrain the client if necessary (for example, if a client is in danger of seriously harming herself or others). This collaboration gives the client as much choice as possible, and keeps the process between therapist and client mutual and predictable.

Developing the treatment frame

The treatment frame refers to the ground rules of therapy. Most clients need to be educated about the expectations of therapy. Mental health professionals must make their expectations and rules of therapy explicit and concrete. Most trauma clients do not have the ability (ego resources) to negotiate the interpersonal world and manage relationships as effectively as they might. They often need help in knowing how to develop mature mutual relationships and how to establish boundaries.

The following therapeutic issues identified by clinicians Chu (1998), Courtois (1999) and Pearlman (2001) — safety, clear expectations, boundaries and disagreements — have been identified as key issues that mental health professionals need to address.

Safety
The personal safety of both client and therapist are the first concern in therapy. Safety issues include:
• attention to living arrangements for women in abusive relationships
• hospitalization for clients who are actively suicidal or need protection from self-harming behaviours
• medication for clients whose depression, anxiety, and sleep problems are debilitating (Pearlman, 2001).

Safety for the therapist includes the risk of danger or harm from a client who re-enacts abuse dynamics. Therapists must maintain that they cannot work if their safety is compromised by threats or actively aggressive behaviour. Serious threats or actions should be grounds for ending therapy or, at least, must be understood and controlled before therapy can continue (Courtois, 1999).

Clear expectations
Clients must be clearly informed of:
• arrangements for fees, billing and payment schedule
• attendance requirements
• procedures for missed appointments
• the length and frequency of sessions.

Consistent and predictable expectations are important in creating safety, because many clients have experienced childhood abuse that included shifting rules and unnamed and inappropriate expectations.

Boundaries
Boundaries are respected and maintained in the following ways:
• The therapist keeps the appointment time and does not miss appointments, start late, reschedule without explanation or run sessions over time.
• Mental health professionals clarify their accessibility and the means of contact outside of the office. For example, some therapists are willing to accept evening and weekend calls, while others are not.
• The relationship between the therapist and client takes place in the office, and there are no dual relationships. This includes general practitioners

(medical doctors) who conduct psychotherapy with patients.* They must refer the patient to another doctor for physical examinations, especially internal examinations. Therapists should not have any social or business relationships with clients.

• Therapists should acknowledge any mistakes and missteps they make. For example, if a client asks a therapist if he or she is tired, distracted or frustrated, the therapist must answer honestly and with care. This helps develop trust and validate the client's perceptions (Saakvitne, Gamble, Pearlman & Lev, 2000).

• Even though the therapist is striving for honesty, boundaries must not be compromised by lapsing into harmful self-disclosure. For example, while admitting to being tired, the therapist should not go into detail about why she or he is not sleeping well, or describe any personal stresses.

Disagreements

• The therapist is authentic and open in the session and invites discussion from clients on the process of therapy, including ongoing assessments of what is working and what is not. Clients are educated to expect that difficulties and disagreements are inevitable in the therapeutic relationship, like all relationships, and that these disagreements should not be treated as signs of failure (Courtois, 1999; Chu, 1998). Rather, clients will learn that conflict and differences can be worked through successfully, resulting in therapeutic gain.

• Clients need to know that they have the right to end therapy at any time, but they also need to be encouraged to try to problem solve or work to resolution. Trauma clients are sensitive to interpersonal cues and often misinterpret and misunderstand such cues. They also may not have had the experience of working through conflicts, so they need to be able to verbalize their concerns and they need to be taught communication and conflict resolution skills (Courtois, 1999).

Transference issues

Many trauma survivors experienced abuse that, by its very nature, includes a violation and disregard for their personal boundaries. Often, they have had

*The education for a medical degree in no way provides training for mental health work or advanced therapeutic skills. To undertake this kind of specialized therapeutic work, general practitioners should have received significant professional training well beyond what is required for a medical degree.

a lifetime of intrusive and blurred boundaries between themselves and others. Mental health professionals are obligated to be scrupulous and acutely aware of their own professional boundaries; they must be aware of their emotional attunement, attachment and availability, as well as of the client's patterns of relating (Courtois, 1999).

Role re-enactments
Trauma clients are known to have intense transference and traumatic role re-enactments. These relational patterns have been well documented and are often easily recognized (the common abuse roles are victim, victimizer, rescuer, and bystander) (Davies & Frawley, 1994). The therapist must learn to recognize these relational dynamics, to avoid participating in them and to help the client understand these dynamics.

Many mental health professionals fall into the role of rescuer when working with a trauma client who is compliant, idealizing and dependent, or one whose behaviour results in the therapist feeling anxious and afraid for the client's well-being. Sometimes, the therapist will wish to protect these clients.

It is generally counter-therapeutic for therapists to try to rescue clients, as this promotes unhealthy dependence, and therapists will eventually feel emotionally stretched and burned out. These therapists may become angry at their client's demands and move from the role of rescuer to victim and, ultimately, to victimizer. As a result of their anger and feelings of incompetence, therapists may become hostile or punitive (Davies & Frawley, 1994). It is up to the therapist to monitor transference and counter-transference responses and to address problematic boundary issues as they occur.

Counter-transference issues
Counter-transference describes the emotional responses and reactions that therapists have about clients. All therapists have emotional responses towards clients; these are a normal and necessary part of therapeutic work. Counter-transference responses with abuse survivors are often complex and intense and can place significant emotional strain on therapists.

Vicarious trauma
Vicarious trauma describes the process by which mental health professionals have their own overwhelming responses to hearing about the terrible details of clients' abuse stories. It is of particular concern for some therapists.

Therapists can experience shock, disbelief, confusion and even a pervasive sense of their own vulnerability (Chu, 1998).

These responses are common, and mental health professionals must develop personal support from friends, family, colleagues, and/or their own therapists. Valuable resources have been developed to help discuss vicarious trauma in mental health professionals (see Resources, p. 187).

Therapist discomfort
Chu (1998) describes how unacknowledged therapist discomfort (frustration, anger, dysphoria) causes counter-transference difficulty, resulting in the use of defence mechanisms. He explains that most therapists would not express overt hostility but may find themselves becoming neglectful or distant.

Some typical behaviours the therapist may use include: failure to follow through with commitments, forgetfulness concerning appointments, habitual lateness, taking phone calls during sessions, excessive note-taking or scheduling appointments in an erratic or unpredictable manner (Chu, 1998).

Managing counter-transference reactions
The nature of mental health professionals' responses and reactions to clients can hold valuable information, depending on how aware therapists are and how they use their reactions to clients in their work. Therapists who notice their feelings, reflect on them and decide upon the most appropriate response to them find that their responses are a useful guide throughout the therapeutic process.

CASE STUDY: COUNTER-TRANSFERENCE REACTIONS

A therapist starts to feel impatient and irritated when her client reports that everyone fails her because all they care about is themselves. The therapist catches herself wanting to confront the client and point out all the times that she has gone out of her way to help her. The therapist realizes that the response she wants to give is therapeutically not a useful one; it is a reaction to her own frustration and feeling unappreciated by this client.

Instead of responding to the client with frustration and irritation, which could hurt and shame the client, the therapist can use empathy and a problem-solving approach:

▶ "I know that many times in your life you have not been protected
or responded to by significant people in your life. I know you are
struggling to trust that friends and people you care about will be
responsive. I wonder what support you need right now and how
I can help you communicate and negotiate that with your friends."

In this example, the therapist's frustration led her to realize that the client's
friends and intimates likely feel similarly frustrated and often may avoid the
client. Instead of responding to the client as if she were whiny and com-
plaining, the therapist decided to respond to the client's distress. In this way,
the therapist empowered the client to consider more effective ways to communicate her needs with people in her life.

Professional support for counter-transference
Generally, mental health professionals need professional support to manage
their counter-transference, including ongoing consultation, continuing
education programs and support from colleagues. Chu (1998) eloquently
explains that therapists need to practise what they preach and seek interpersonal support and connection in times of stress. Trauma clients learn from
their therapists' examples. Having a therapist model how to resolve a relational impasse, therefore, is an invaluable lesson in the therapeutic process.

VALIDATION AND EMPATHIC ATTUNEMENT
It is critical for the mental health professional to validate the client's emotional responses and reactions to her early abuse experience as well as to
normalize the creative adaptations she has developed to survive the trauma.
To do this, a therapist has to understand the long-term effects of abuse and
trauma and the adaptive function of "symptoms" of this abuse (see Chapter
8: The Importance of Carrying Out Psychoeducation with Clients).

> Most importantly, clinicians developing treatment approaches for trauma
> work would almost all agree that **empathic attunement** is an essential,
> and possibly the most critical, element of the healing process (Courtois,
> 1999, Chu, 1998).

Chu (1998) points out that trauma survivors typically deny, minimize, blame themselves and express shame about what was done to them during the abuse, as well as about what they needed to do to survive these experiences. Mental health professionals can play an essential role in helping to shift these feelings of shame by diligently working to reframe the self-blaming and criticism that survivors may use to talk about themselves (or other abuse survivors).

Developing compassion for herself may involve encouraging a client to remember the vulnerability and relative powerlessness inherent in being a child. It may also involve respectfully acknowledging her attempts to master and cope with the abusive situation.

CASE STUDY: VALIDATION

A client believes she is responsible for the abuse that happened to her, because when she was a child her perpetrator told her she was "sexy." Her guilt is intensified by the fact that she liked the attention paid to her by her perpetrator.

The mental health professional can point out to the client that:

▶ "You were a seven-year-old little girl who responded positively to being told she was pretty. That does not mean that you were in any way responsible for your offender's sexual abuse of you. Not only have you suffered from the hurt and betrayal that someone you trusted and cared for sexually violated you. You also have suffered with shame and self-hate because you believed you were responsible when your perpetrator blamed you for the abuse, by saying that you were sexy and you turned him on."

Many therapists express frustration that survivors repeatedly return to the same self-blaming and self-hating sentiments.

It is important to remember that these self-blaming beliefs (schemas) have been in place for many women since early childhood, and our victim-blaming society helps to reinforce these beliefs. They are, therefore, both deeply entrenched and socially reinforced.

Therapists may also have to reframe and repeat the same non-blaming, empathic responses many times, and from many different perspectives, before some clients will be able to acknowledge and integrate these new messages. This may be a protracted part of the therapeutic work and requires ongoing reinforcement.

EMPOWERING CLIENTS TO MAKE CHANGES

While it is critical to validate survivors' feelings of pain and despair, it is also important to ensure that they not lose sight of the potential for and possibility of change in their lives. Clients should know that the therapeutic process is intended to help them develop the skills and resources they need to experience feelings of self-efficacy and control — and to reduce their suffering.

Mental health professionals must remain committed to the belief that clients are not helpless to change their reactions to their own internal processes. If mental health professionals act as if they are the authorities who best know what their clients need, they inadvertently recreate a paternalistic and disempowering therapeutic relationship. This often brings up a client's feelings of danger, betrayal and shame.

Although many clients often feel overwhelmed and helpless, there are ways to achieve mastery over these feelings. The therapist must guide clients through the process of recognizing how feelings from the past get re-experienced in the present, so clients can disengage the past from the present and develop new coping responses.

Trauma survivors will feel safest when they are actively participating and making decisions in the process of therapy. Their empowerment is accomplished by therapists who:
• set mutual goals
• provide information on the therapeutic process
• guide and help clients in establishing the pace of therapy
• invite clients to offer feedback on their experience of therapy.

In adopting this approach, therapists show respect for the autonomy of their clients.

Many therapists struggle to find the balance between demonstrating respect for a client's intense emotional pain and staying convinced that the client needs to develop different coping behaviours and responses. This balance of empathy and responsibility is critical within therapeutic work.

> Empathy without a belief that the client is able to make changes to help herself results in disempowering the client. On the other hand, therapists who emphasize change and responsibility without expressing empathy for their client's struggle in making these changes may be perceived by the client as critical and blaming.

CASE STUDY: BALANCING EMPATHY AND RESPONSIBILITY

A woman who experienced abandonment and neglect as a child flies into a rage whenever someone is late to meet her. The therapist needs to validate and empathize with the feelings of fear this triggers while, at the same time, emphasize that the survivor is vividly re-experiencing feelings of being abandoned from the past, as if she were being abandoned in the present.

It is understandable that this woman feels such an intense response because of what it brings up from her childhood. But she also needs to recognize that her reactions are now those of an adult and are out of proportion to the incident that is upsetting her.

Rather than acting on these feelings, she can learn to recognize them for what they are, and then choose how to respond. For example, she can soothe herself by using a comforting visualization, she can cognitively reframe what happened and remind herself that that was then and this is now, or she can take time out to detach from her intense reactions.

A possible empathic response from the therapist might sound something like:

▶ "I can tell how afraid and anxious you feel whenever you think someone is not going to meet you when they say they would. It makes you feel abandoned and forgotten. These feelings are so intense for you, because they resonate with what you felt as a child. It is important for you to recognize that as an adult you have choices available to you that you did not have as a child. With practice, you can learn to recognize and interrupt these old patterns of responding."

Women will be able to feel a greater sense of self-efficacy, control and mastery in their lives as they learn to make changes in the way they respond to upsetting events, and as the therapist validates their feelings.

Recognizing and naming client strengths

A therapist will often assess a client's vulnerabilities and symptoms as the starting point for therapeutic treatment without *also* assessing the client's strengths and abilities. This type of approach is not only disempowering, but it also does not offer hope. Moreover, it can set the stage for survivors to feel dependent, helpless and stigmatized.

One of the most powerful ways to show respect is to recognize and emphasize a woman's positive attributes, rather than simply associate her with a series of symptoms and deficits. This highlighting of strengths will help the survivor move beyond a sense of stigmatization and shame.

IDENTIFYING CLIENTS' STRENGTHS MEANS RECOGNIZING THE SURVIVOR'S:
- skills, talents and abilities
- resources
- resilience and achievements.

Some clinicians have developed methods to assess and integrate their clients' strengths as part of both the initial assessment and the ongoing therapy. Meichenbaum (1994) acknowledges clients' strengths throughout therapy by using a number of empathic and validating statements. For example, after a client discusses any achievement (e.g., graduating from school, solving a problem with her children), the therapist can respond by saying: "You accomplished (X) in spite of (whatever negative life event she has mentioned)."

Maxine Harris' book *Trauma Recovery and Empowerment* (1998) includes a self-esteem achievement chart as a therapeutic tool. On one side of the chart, the client lists five things in her life that she feels good about. She then rates each of these from one to 10, in terms of the strength of the positive feeling. Examples of experiences she feels good about might include the birth of a child; graduating from high school, community college or university; staying sober; and holding a job. Less obvious gains can also be recognized as achievements, such as making a positive change, expressing herself directly or recognizing a trauma response without acting on it.

Often clients will not recognize their own resources and strengths, and, if asked to list them, they may feel either inadequate or ashamed. It is helpful if the therapist, together with the client, extracts the client's strengths from her description of how she coped or responded to different situations in her daily life.

An example of highlighting interpersonal strengths is helping a woman see her accomplishments in the face of the abuse she experienced, by saying something like:

► **"You were able to *not* accept [the perpetrator's] definition of you [use the client's own example; e.g., "that you were useless"] and, in fact, you provided good care and support to your children."**

The clinical tool on the text page (Identifying client strengths – A tool for clinicians) can help mental health professionals draw out and highlight clients' strengths and abilities.

Here is a clinical example of how this can be effectively used with a client who blames herself for all of the problems and difficulties she experiences.

First, the therapist and client identify that "empathy for others" is one on the client's personal strengths. To apply this strength, the client is asked what kind of empathic response she would offer to another woman who blames herself. The client is then asked to imagine hearing that same empathic response directed back at her.

Identifying client strengths — A tool for clinicians

Potential Strengths

• ability to have perspective and see alternative viewpoints

• ability to have empathy for self and/or others

• ability to set appropriate boundaries in relationships with others

• willpower and initiative

• awareness of own psychological needs

• sense of humour

• insight, ability to be introspective

• ability to establish mature relationships with others

• ability to make self-protective judgments

Client Strengths

Identify areas of strength you see in this client:

1. _____

2. _____

3. _____

Application of Client's Strengths

In addition to sharing this list of strengths with the client, how else can you and the client discuss applying these strengths to increase symptom management and stabilization?

1. for example, _____

2. _____

3. _____

(Saakvitne, Gamble, Pearlman & Lev. Adapted from *Risking Connection: A Training Curriculum for Working with Survivors of Childhood Abuse* with permission from Sidran Press. Copyright 2000. The full *Risking Connection* curriculum is available from Sidran Press: www.sidran.org or 410.825.8888.)

RESPECTFUL ENGAGEMENT / ACTIVE FACILITATION

For many survivors, the context of their abuse was one of silence and secrecy. Sometimes the silence was the speechless actions of their perpetrator sexually abusing them in the night. For others who grew up in the context of neglect and abandonment, the silence was not being told they were loved, valued and deserving of protection. There is also the larger silence of years of not speaking about the atrocities committed against them and the silence of a society that only recently and inadequately acknowledges childhood abuse and neglect.

When a therapist sits with a survivor and hears her despair and pain, and remains silent, many survivors will feel even more fear and shame. Some therapeutic engagement with this material is needed.

It is important for therapists to:

• Actively express their reactions so that clients understand how the therapist is thinking and feeling about what the client is disclosing. Make a direct statement, such as: "I now understand why you feel [specify feeling]." Or say: "What a horrible experience to have lived through." This kind of statement reflects the therapist's empathic reactions, whereas simply asking the client, "How did this experience make you feel?" asks her to disclose more information without receiving any reassuring feedback.

• Be familiar with reframing statements and normalizing comments (see Chapter 8: The Importance of Carrying Out Psychoeducation with Clients). For example, if a woman tells the therapist she never tells anyone about her past experiences of abuse, a normalizing response would be: "That is a way you try to keep yourself protected from being hurt by other people's lack of knowledge about these difficult experiences."

• Know themselves and know how they feel and think about abuse. This will enable them to be present and self-aware in the therapeutic process, and to be engaged and empathic without being intrusive. Clients experience questions as intrusive if they are asked in a demanding way or with a tone of judgment or disbelief. Nor should the client be burdened with self-revelations or extreme responses from the mental health professional.

> It is critically important that mental health professionals avoid making the following mistakes when discussing trauma and abuse with a client:
> • When validating the client's experience of violation, don't make sweeping statements about abuse. For example, many clients blame themselves, and believe they actively participated or were complicit in the abuse. As a result, they may interpret statements, such as "abuse is wrong," to mean they have done something bad. Offer more nuanced responses to explain the harm of abuse, such as:

▶ "What was done to you was wrong."

"Children can never consent to sex with an adult."

"Children often accommodate unwanted sexual acts as a way to survive what was done to them."

> • Therapists should be careful not to burden clients with their own revelations or with strong or extreme responses. The balance is important to find. It is inappropriate to express anger at the person who perpetrated the abuse. Many survivors haven't come to terms with their own anger; they may feel alienated by this response from their therapist and may feel a need to protect the perpetrator.

PART III
Tools and Strategies

While people working in the field emphasize that clients must learn essential coping skills to benefit from trauma treatment, the literature doesn't adequately or specifically explain what these specific skills are. Nor does it offer much in the way of practical strategies or clinical interventions needed to do this therapeutic work.

Part III of this guidebook offers information about the process of conducting psychotherapy with trauma survivors, as well as techniques and interventions to be used in first stage trauma treatment.

The exercises are designed to allow mental health professionals develop a repertoire of effective and concrete clinical tools and strategies for first stage trauma treatment. They may need to be tailored to the individual client's needs, and they may need to be used many times.

CHAPTER 8
The Importance of Carrying Out Psychoeducation with Clients

This chapter emphasizes the importance of psychoeducation in trauma therapy. It addresses:
• general issues of psychoeducation
• making the connection between childhood abuse and trauma
• normalizing client responses to trauma
• what information to include in psychoeducation.

Chapters 9 and 10 outline the specifics of this information and methods of delivery.

CHAPTER 8
The Importance of Carrying Out Psychoeducation with Clients

In this book, the term psychoeducation describes the process of working with clients to explain and make visible the nature of psychological processes.

Psychoeducation about post-traumatic stress and the psychobiological responses of trauma survivors is a critical component of first stage trauma treatment. Education about post-traumatic stress creates hope in clients — if their problem "has a name," it is understood and can be treated (Meichenbaum, 1994).

> **THE PURPOSE OF PSYCHOEDUCATION IS NOT SIMPLY TO CONVEY INFORMATION BUT ALSO TO:**
> - instill hope
> - engender meaning
> - help construct new narratives
> - control post-traumatic stress responses.

This chapter is divided into two parts. The first addresses general approaches to ongoing psychoeducation with clients. The second part covers the treatment interventions and coping strategies that clients can learn and use to help control their trauma responses.

GENERAL ISSUES OF PSYCHOEDUCATION
Psychoeducation typically relies on cognitive-behavioural approaches. The cognitive component includes setting out a framework for the psycho-

education and creating approaches to manage and stabilize trauma responses. The behavioural component consists of learning and practising interventions until the desired therapeutic goals are achieved.

The psychoeducational aspects of first stage trauma work should be woven throughout the sessions, directed by and relating to what the client is discussing and processing.

Pace and timing

When introducing information about how people respond to traumatic events, the pace and timing should be tailored to the individual client. This ensures the client knows that the therapist has heard her individual experience, and has understood her particular emotional distress. Some therapists audiotape these sessions and give the client a copy to refer to later in the therapeutic work.

Listening and normalizing

Psychoeducation does not mean that the therapist spends several sessions lecturing clients in a didactic manner, or illustrates concepts through diagrams and handouts. Instead, the therapist should listen carefully to the client's story and normalize and validate the client's reactions to the traumatic events she has experienced.

The therapist can then educate the client about the bio-psycho-social dimensions of post-traumatic stress and the physiological impact of having experienced traumatic events.

Understanding client reactions

Therapists must understand these concepts, and be able to use and explain them, to help survivors understand typical and understandable reactions.

For example, when a survivor minimizes or denies the importance of her abusive experience, the therapist can point out that many children survived by pretending that the abuse was not happening to them. Often, denial about abuse developed in childhood is still present into adulthood. Many survivors are emotionally constricted and have spent a lifetime minimizing their abuse. As a result, they may not even initially report having had abusive experiences.

However, an informed therapist will be able to infer from the client's abuse history and current responses and symptoms that she probably had a psychically overwhelming experience and that her psychological defences are still protecting her from fully acknowledging that experience. In cases where clients had childhoods of neglect and deprivation, they likely cannot name what they did not receive. For example, they will not be able to identify that they did not develop secure attachments. A history of troubled and difficult relationships will, however, offer the therapist the first clues.

Client readiness
Not all clients will want or need this psychoeducational information, or they may not be ready for it, or at least not all of it. A survivor may not be able to construct a narrative of her childhood experiences for herself, or even have the language to discuss her experiences.

This doesn't mean that the therapist retreats from conducting the essential work of first stage trauma therapy. Mental health professionals must, most importantly, determine how the client is functioning in her everyday life. A carefully paced model of containment and skill building can be carried out with survivors, regardless of their ability to acknowledge or express the magnitude of earlier abuse or neglect. Survivors may not feel the impact of what has happened to them, but their skills deficits will most likely be evident. The therapist can gently start incorporating the connection between past abuse and neglect and the current difficulties into the psychoeducational therapy.

MAKING THE CONNECTION BETWEEN CHILDHOOD ABUSE AND TRAUMA

To ignore the role of abusive experiences is to tacitly collude in abuse survivors' denial of the impact of the abuse, as well as in their erroneous beliefs of personal defectiveness (Chu 1998, p. 81).

Although Chu advises against probing past abuse in first stage trauma treatment, he argues that acknowledging the central role of abuse is essential.

> It doesn't make sense to offer a decontextualized account of trauma without first acknowledging the survivors' own experience. This acknowledgment of the role of the traumatic experience helps survivors understand that many of their current difficulties are normal adaptive responses to overwhelming life experiences of abuse or neglect.

Therapists must reiterate that although clients must ultimately shoulder the responsibility of the recovery process, they are not responsible for the abuse itself. Identifying and naming an experience as abuse or neglect is not an easy task, nor is it a discussion that can be covered in one session. Most often, the therapist will have to review this issue repeatedly and over time, and present it from a variety of different perspectives.

NORMALIZATION

Normalizing the coping strategies survivors use to deal with traumatic effects is an important element of trauma treatment.

Most therapists working from a trauma framework promote the idea of reframing "negative symptoms" as:
• healthy adaptations or responses
• coping strategies
• self-protections.

Many trauma survivors tend to have judged themselves harshly, and have misinterpreted their reactions and symptoms as "abnormal" and/or "crazy." Often they have been pathologized by others. They are relieved, therefore, to learn that their reactions are not only normal, but also that they are predictable responses and that many other people have suffered in similar ways after experiencing traumatic events.

> In working with women who have experienced abuse-related trauma, it is important to emphasize that nothing is wrong with them — rather, something wrong has happened to them.
>
> It is also crucial to convey that is not unusual to "feel crazy" or believe that one is "losing one's mind." Such feelings are an indication that important responses to the trauma need to be worked through, and that

> these responses may manifest themselves in a variety of physical or mental health symptoms.

Many of us have seen films or other media depictions of such experiences as a war veteran reliving (having a flashback of) the horrors of a battle. However, other common effects of post-traumatic stress, such as dissociation, hyperarousal and emotional numbing resulting from childhood abuse, typically don't get depicted or discussed. These responses are often frightening and bewildering for survivors. Moreover, because they already feel so ashamed and stigmatized, abuse survivors are often hesitant to discuss some of the more disturbing responses they are experiencing. It is important, therefore, to normalize these experiences and explain that these responses are a predictable part of psychological trauma.

The mental health professional must determine what symptoms make the client feel most distressed and:
• give information about these reactions
• normalize and de-stigmatize responses by relating them to the universal effects of trauma.

The following case study is an example of working therapeutically to normalize a woman's response to trauma.

CASE STUDY: NORMALIZING RESPONSES TO TRAUMA

Whenever a client named Sarah was distressed, she saw fairies that looked like Tinker Bell from *Peter Pan*. These tiny, fluttery beings were so beautiful and so caring that they distracted her from the immediacy of her experience.

Once, while watching a documentary about a sexual abuse survivor, Sarah became enthralled by a beautiful painting of a fairy made by the abuse survivor. Sarah mentioned to a friend who was going to view the same documentary that she should watch for this beautiful fairy painting.

The friend later reported to Sarah that the painting was not of a fairy, but rather was one of the most disturbing depictions that she had ever seen of a woman's experience of being molested. As a result, Sarah believed she was psychotic and became extremely secretive and ashamed about her experience of sometimes seeing fairies. Rather than serving an essential soothing function, fairies took on a terrifying new meaning. Her important adaptive source of self-protection was now lost.

Sarah learned from her therapist, who was trained in working with sexual abuse and in working with people dealing with post-traumatic stress, that fairies helped her cope with her overwhelming experiences of abuse.

Later on in therapy, Sarah recalled that, as a child, she had had a Peter Pan lamp by her bedside that she would focus on while she was being sexually abused. Fairies gave her a place to go when the present was too unbearable to tolerate. Fairies were a special gift that enabled her to survive, not an indication of mental illness. In this way, Sarah realized that she had learned as a child to use the fairies from the Peter Pan lamp to comfort herself and to escape and survive the overwhelming feelings brought on by the violation of being sexually abused. Understood in this way, Sarah no longer felt "crazy" and "psychotic" for seeing fairies, but understood their origin and their function.

Normalizing post-traumatic stress responses can help shift core abuse-related beliefs and cognitions that may have reinforced the client's symptoms of depression, anxiety or avoidance. Psychoeducation about trauma can provide significant relief in and of itself, which, in turn, empowers trauma survivors.

THE FOCUS OF PSYCHOEDUCATIONAL WORK

In first stage trauma treatment, most direct work should be educational and cognitive. This includes giving survivors information about the immediate impact of trauma as well as its long-lasting after-effects.

Survivors need to understand the range and complexity of post-traumatic stress responses, including the dimensions of both simple post-traumatic stress, complex post-traumatic stress, and the typical responses and adaptations that survivors develop.

Psychoeducation includes information about abuse and neglect, and the resulting trauma responses. However, the complexity of trauma responses and the therapeutic work involved to resolve them will not be fully understood unless clients also understand the developmental issues associated with complex post-traumatic stress. Most people who develop complex post-traumatic stress were exposed to chronic stressors (abuse, deprivation and/or neglect) in childhood, resulting in pervasive effects on their social and personality development. The age at which the traumatic event occurs also shapes subsequent adaptation patterns.

Most clients, therefore, eventually need to understand how abuse and neglect shaped their development and responses as children, as well as their responses in adulthood. Through this lens, they can reinterpret their lives in a way that is meaningful and coherent and begin developing compassion and connection for the children they once were.

CHAPTER 9
Explaining Simple Post-Traumatic Stress Responses to Clients

This chapter contains information to help therapists explain simple post-traumatic stress responses to clients, including:

- what simple post traumatic stress is
- how to identify simple post traumatic stress
- the ways people survive trauma
- the differences between simple and complex post-traumatic stress
- re-experiencing phenomena
- avoiding and numbing
- hyperarousal.

CHAPTER 9
Explaining Simple
Post-Traumatic Stress
Responses to Clients

Before clients can start to understand their specific trauma reactions and symptoms, they need to understand that their childhood and adult experiences of abuse and neglect have discernible biological, psychological and social (bio-psycho-social) consequences. This begins with explaining what trauma itself is.

The following section contains information therapists can use to explain trauma to their clients. It is written to give mental health professionals a sense of the way this information can be conveyed to clients and, in places, provides examples of actual scripts. In most cases, however, mental health professionals will have to use their clinical judgment about the best way to distill and present this information to clients — based on where clients are in the therapy process and tailored to their individual pacing and information needs.

EXPLAINING TRAUMA
Explain to clients that:

▶ **Trauma refers to the effects of severe neglect, emotional, physical and/or sexual abuse, as well as physical and sexual assault.**

A good working definition of trauma is as follows:

A traumatic experience is an event that continues to exert negative effects on thinking (cognition), feeling (affect) and behaviour, long after the event is in the past.

The terms "trauma response" or "traumatic stress" describe the effects of traumatic experiences.

Explain to clients that:

▶ • People react to traumatic experiences in vastly different ways.
- Some of the responses might be obvious to you, such as intrusive memories or panic attacks. Other responses, such as feeling numb and empty, are subtle and harder to identify.
- These responses may continue for years following the traumatic event(s). In some cases, responses may subside and return later, which is often the case with survivors of childhood abuse.
- Sometimes the experience of an adult sexual or physical assault can trigger trauma responses from childhood — responses that you were unaware were still unresolved.

The trauma response — reacting to abuse and other harmful events

It is important to explain to clients that whether an event is considered traumatic is determined by their subjective experience. A traumatic event or situation creates psychological trauma when it overwhelms the person's perceived ability to cope, and leaves that person fearing that she will be hurt or killed or that she will lose her mind.

Explain to clients that trauma comes in many forms, and people cope in different ways. There are, however, similarities in the experiences and the patterns of responses depending on:
- whether it was a single traumatic incident versus repeated experiences
- the age when the trauma occurred
- the relationship to the perpetrator.

Repeated early childhood trauma is especially damaging in the ways that it interrupts emotional, psychological and physiological development. These traumatic events (especially those repeatedly experienced in childhood) affect a survivor's brain, mind, spirit, and body. During traumatic experience(s), people do whatever they can to survive.

EXPLAINING WAYS OF SURVIVING TRAUMA

Clients need to know that one of the ways in which trauma is processed is in terms of the "fight or flight" reaction.

The "fight-or-flight" reaction

Explain to clients that:

▶ when in danger or threatened, our bodies are programmed to have a fight-or-flight response. When people are unable to actually fight or take flight — as is the case with most children who are abused and many women who are assaulted by their male partners — they are both emotionally and physically trapped.

Coping behaviours and adaptations

Then explain how the fight-or-flight reaction leads to coping behaviours and adaptations:

▶ Unable to take flight or fight, survivors must find other ways to handle these overwhelming experiences. Some of the coping responses learned include dissociating, going numb or disconnecting. These coping behaviours typically do what they are supposed to — they help people survive. However, when the abuse is prolonged and repeated, these coping behaviours result in psychological and physiological changes or adaptations, such as changes in perception, feelings and behaviours, that have long-term consequences. For example, some of these responses keep the body on high alert for danger (arousal and hypervigilance) or disconnected and numb to avoid feeling pain.

Eventually, these adaptations become limited in their effectiveness. As a result, an important first stage in your healing is to see what coping responses you developed to survive and assess whether the responses are interfering with the quality of your present-day life.

Family influence

The next step is to explore family influence. Explain to clients that:

▶ The type of family you came from can also influence the long-term impact of traumatic experiences. Having someone you are bonded with, are loved by and feel safe with provides comfort and reassurance. This type of attachment also provides a buffer from the abuse.

Additionally, people from close, loving families develop internal resources and skills that help them overcome traumatic stress responses. They learn skills such as how to calm themselves down quickly even when something very upsetting happens to them.

On the other hand, people from families that are distant, frightening and unpredictable do not have an emotional buffer from the abuse. Even worse, they may have been punished for being upset or angry, or rejected when they needed comfort.

People from these families often were not able to develop the skills or internal abilities to calm or soothe themselves. So, there is a "double whammy" — overwhelming experiences of abuse and the absence of comfort or solace.

Abuse survivors who grew up in unhealthy family environments face greater challenges in their healing processes. They have to develop, strengthen or rebuild fundamental skills that they need to fully function and heal.

The positive and hopeful part of this is that with tremendous patience and endurance, and the help of a skilled and experienced therapist, the necessary skills to overcome trauma responses and symptoms can be developed.

Healing processes

Clients need to know that healing involves two main processes:

► 1. Identifying the coping behaviours and adaptations that you developed to survive the abuse.
2. Developing tools and strategies to improve your coping and help you overcome the disturbing trauma responses or adaptations that still plague you.

EXPLAINING SIMPLE POST-TRAUMATIC STRESS RESPONSES

Clients need to learn that trauma can change a person's development when it disrupts emotion, consciousness, memory, sense of self, attachment to others and relationships. Traumatic experiences alter the functioning of the central nervous system as well as general physiological functioning. These changes in functioning are often referred to as "symptoms," or symptom clusters, particularly when they are given a medical diagnosis, such as post-traumatic stress disorder

Simple PTSD is distinguished by three distinct symptom clusters.

The Three Symptom Clusters of Simple PTSD

THREE SYMPTOM CLUSTERS FORM A COHERENT SYNDROME REFERRED TO AS SIMPLE POST-TRAUMATIC STRESS DISORDER. THESE CLUSTERS ARE:

1. Re-experiencing phenomena — this includes reliving the event through recurring nightmares, flashbacks or other intrusive images that "pop" into one's head at any time.
2. Avoiding/numbing responses — this involves avoiding reminders of the event, including places, people, thoughts or feelings. People who experience these responses become emotionally numb, withdraw from friends and family, and lose interest in everyday activities.
3. Hyper-arousal responses — this includes being chronically on guard at all times, including irritability or sudden anger, difficulty sleeping, lack of concentration, being overly alert or easily startled.

EXPLAINING THE THREE RESPONSE CLUSTERS OF SIMPLE POST-TRAUMATIC STRESS

Re-experiencing phenomena
Explain to clients that intrusive thoughts or ruminations, flashbacks and nightmares are all considered "re-experiencing" phenomena.

- Intrusive thoughts and ruminations are experienced as a constant replay in the mind of the most awful moments of the traumatic experience.
- Flashbacks are sudden, intrusive and vivid re-experiencing of traumatic experiences. The re-experiencing will appear to come out of nowhere, making the person feel out of control. A flashback may involve some or all of the senses; it may be experienced as smells, tastes, bodily sensations, sights and sounds. These sensory memories can be so vivid that a woman may be unaware of her actual surroundings.

> • Nightmares may contain scenes of the actual events or symbolic rep-
> resentations of the original trauma, in which the emotional feelings of
> the original experience are recreated.
>
> Flashbacks, nightmares and ruminations are the brain's attempt to
> make sense of and integrate the traumatic experience — they are the
> brain's attempt to heal itself.

Avoiding and numbing responses

Clients need to understand that traumatized people, faced with difficulties in controlling their emotions, typically expend energy avoiding distressing feelings. They may report feeling "dead to the world."

This emotional numbing can be part of their everyday life. It can be expressed as depression or as dissociative states. Whereas intrusive symptoms occur in response to specific stimuli after being traumatized, many survivors report that they no longer take pleasure in activities they once enjoyed. They feel that they just "go through the motions" of everyday living.

Explain to clients that:

▶ Avoidant responses include efforts to avoid thoughts, feelings or conversations about the trauma. Numbing describes the way people blunt their feelings to make them more manageable.

AVOIDING AND NUMBING RESPONSES HELP THE MIND:
- take a "time out"
- "pace" itself, to avoid dealing with overwhelming stress all at once
- restrict the range of feelings dealt with at any one moment
- withdraw from distressing information at a time when a person can-not confront or assimilate the information
- avoid relationships and the feelings that intimacy may evoke. Being intimate may bring up the fear of feeling too much.

(Meichenbaum, 1994)

Hyperarousal responses

Explain to clients that:

▶ "Hyperarousal" describes a state of heightened and chronic arousal characterized by:
- insomnia
- irritability
- difficulty concentrating
- hypervigilance
- exaggerated startle responses.

"Hypervigilance" is constant heightened awareness of your surroundings to protect against potential harm or danger (i.e., feeling the need to be on guard all the time).

Hyperarousal and hypervigilance are the after-effects of your brain being "turned on" to sense danger. These are predictable responses to being placed in dangerous and hurtful situations.

In particular, fear is an emotion that alerts people to pay attention, so that they can act/respond to the situation. Chronic arousal interferes with your ability to use your emotions to help you make decisions about how to act.

Children and adults with hyperarousal also tend to have sleep problems. This is for two reasons: they are unable to quiet themselves enough to go to sleep, and they deliberately wake themselves up to avoid having traumatic nightmares.

CHAPTER 10
Explaining Complex Post-Traumatic Stress Responses to Clients

This chapter contains information to help mental health professionals explain complex PTSR to clients. It also helps therapists explain the six dimensions of complex post-traumatic stress:
- affect dysregulation, affect modulation and self-soothing
- dissociation and changes in consciousness
- changes in self-perception
- disturbances in relationships
- somatization
- alterations in systems of meaning.

CHAPTER 10
Explaining Complex Post-Traumatic Stress Responses to Clients

In addition to explaining the nature of simple post-traumatic stress responses to clients, therapists need to explain complex post-traumatic stress responses and offer information on the bio-psycho-social development of these difficulties.

The general distinction is that simple PTSR typically develops after a single-event trauma. On the other hand, people are more likely to experience complex PTSR if their abuse or neglect experiences occurred early in life, if the abuse was prolonged, and if it was perpetrated by one's own caregivers. Complex PTSR can develop as the result of chronic adult experiences as well (e.g., women in prolonged relationships where they were battered).

> Many trauma clients will have *both* simple and complex post-traumatic stress responses and adaptations.

There are six dimensions to complex PTSR:
1. affect dysregulation
2. dissociation and changes in consciousness
3. changes in self -perception
4. disturbances in relationships
5. somatization
6. alterations in systems of meaning.

First stage trauma treatment primarily focuses on:
• affect dysregulation

- dissociation
- changes in self-perception.

However, it is still important to offer clients an overview and outline of the six dimensions of the phenomenon of complex post-traumatic stress.

EXPLAINING THE DIMENSIONS OF COMPLEX POST-TRAUMATIC STRESS RESPONSES
Explain to clients that:

▶ People with complex post-traumatic stress may have some of the following problems:

1. Affect dysregulation
Trauma survivors may have problems with their ability to regulate their emotions. This is known as affect dysregulation. They may have emotional outbursts, emotional swings or impulsiveness. People with affect dysregulation sometimes self-harm, have problems with eating and may have problems with alcohol or other drugs.

2. Dissociation and changes in consciousness
Some survivors may find it hard to stay present without becoming dissociative (spaced out), depersonalized or preoccupied with the abuse.

3. Changes in self-perception
Many survivors perceive themselves as helpless, shameful, guilty, stigmatized, alone and/or feel full of self-blame.

4. Disturbances in relationships
Often survivors find it challenging to have relationships with others without feeling threatened and distrustful. As a result, they may isolate themselves or withdraw from people. They may have had experiences of revictimization; that is, they have been abused by more than one person in their lifetime.

5. Somatization
Survivors often have persistent physical complaints that are hard to diagnose or treat, such as headaches, irritable bowel syndrome or chronic pain.

6. Alterations in systems of meaning

Survivors may be unable to find meaning, faith, hopefulness, and a sense of the future in their lives.

> Clients especially need to have the concepts of affect dysregulation and dissociation explained to them, because these responses are bewildering and frightening to most abuse survivors.

Because dealing with affect dysregulation is central to first stage trauma treatment, the following information also offers examples of the most typical ways it is manifested (e.g., self-harming behaviour, eating disorders, etc.).

EXPLAINING AFFECT DYSREGULATION

Affect dysregulation is considered one of the most challenging aspects of complex PTSR. This is because survivors have such great difficulty calming themselves, and many use extreme measures, such as self-injury, substance use, maladaptive eating, dissociation or risk-taking behaviours, in attempts to manage their emotions. Helping survivors learn to regulate their emotions is often a central focus of trauma treatment.

Three primary therapeutic strategies are used to treat affect dysregulation. These are:

1. psychoeducation
2. providing a contained, predictable therapeutic relationship
3. teaching skills and strategies so clients can develop internal resources to modulate emotion.

> Self-regulation is the ability to modulate or balance physiological arousal (i.e., to have all of one's emotional feelings within relatively comfortable limits). The loss of or deficiency in the ability to self-regulate the intensity of feelings and impulses is called affect dysregulation. This is one of the most far-reaching effects of trauma and neglect and perhaps the most difficult issue for the client.

Explaining affect modulation and self-soothing

It is useful for clients to learn how children modulate their physiological responses to emotion by being soothed or engaged with when they are upset. Survivors did not generally have opportunities to internalize a comforting parent figure, so they typically need to develop and practise specific skills to increase their internal capacity to modulate affect.

To normalize and give a context for why trauma survivors lack this capacity, therapists must educate clients on these developmental processes.

One technique for this is to tell clients the story of the Dog on the Beach.

EXAMPLE: DOG ON THE BEACH

A child is at the beach with her parent when a big, black dog runs towards her barking loudly. The child is scared and runs to her parent for protection. When a child is frightened, what does a protective adult do to help the child manage the experience? The adult reassures the child through comforting touch, and she holds the child to let her know she is safe and to help her feel her body. The adult gives words to the experience, naming feelings, context, and reassurance: "You were frightened when that big dog barked at you. It was scary. It's all right. She won't hurt you. I'm here and will keep you safe." This process teaches a child to identify her feelings, to understand the events that evoked the feelings, and to acknowledge resources for safety and support. Over time and many repetitions a child internalizes the adult's words and soothing presence and can reassure and comfort herself in many situations.

(Saakvitne et al., adapted with permission from The Sidran Press. Copyright 2000.)

Explain to clients that:

▶ Many abuse survivors have had two significant difficulties to cope with:
  • the overwhelming arousal of abuse
  • the absence of adequate soothing and comforting.

That is why trauma survivors sometimes struggle with feeling emotionally constricted or numb while, at other times, they feel flooded with emotion. This can be overcome by learning techniques that help regulate arousal, by learning to put words to your experiences and feelings, and by being offered reassurance.

Explaining coping

The ability to effectively tolerate and cope with strong emotions is an important developmental achievement that is often disrupted in trauma survivors. Instead, survivors of child abuse and neglect often develop coping mechanisms to "switch off" their feelings.

SOME OF THESE COPING MECHANISMS ARE:

- emotional numbing
- denial
- fragmentation of thoughts
- disconnection from bodily feelings.

These coping mechanisms are defences that survivors use to protect themselves from being overwhelmed with feelings and realizations, and from seeing themselves as vulnerable to others in relationships.

However, these mechanisms rarely provide the soothing and balance that survivors require. Instead, survivors often end up alternating between extreme dissociation or constriction and extreme hyperarousal, where they feel flooded and overwhelmed by experiencing an excessive emotional response.

Explain to clients that:

▶   The inability to modulate feelings can result in:
  - self-harming behaviour
  - eating disorders
  - substance use problems
  - a pattern of chaotic relationships
  - symptoms of anxiety, depression or dissociation
  - an unstable sense of self.

These behaviours are all external attempts to self-regulate feelings and internal states. It is often difficult for survivors to give up these self-harming behaviours because they often work, if only temporarily, to ease the disturbing arousal.

If your trauma clients use any of the following coping mechanisms, you can select which information is relevant for your purposes.

Explaining self-harm

Many people (including professionals, therapists and even the survivors themselves) don't understand why survivors harm themselves. This is partly because there is no one reason, as the behaviour serves different functions for different women. Some women may harm themselves to self-soothe, or to relieve a build-up of tension, or both. Some may self-harm to punish themselves and others. And some may self-harm to communicate their distress to therapists or caregivers or to regulate intense and overwhelming feelings.

Therapists must be able to collaborate with trauma clients to determine the function of the self-harming behaviour. However, because self-harming behaviour is often related to attempts to regulate affect, it has been included in this section of the guidebook.

Explain to clients that:

▶ **Many women who self-harm discover that they do it to relieve emotional tension. This tension is often related to the experiences of trauma in early life and not having anyone there to comfort and reassure you. The emotional tension can become intolerable. Women often say they could not find any means to help control these feelings.**

No one can tolerate unending emotional arousal or tension. It is normal and understandable that someone feeling this ongoing tension would try to get relief any way possible. The self-harming behaviour often relieves the tension and helps create a change in mood.

This relief doesn't last, because eventually, without knowing other means of comforting oneself and regulating emotional states, the level of tension and arousal builds up again and women explain that they need to self-harm again.

One of the most important elements in therapy is to make sense of the meanings the self-harm behaviour has for you. The role of

therapy is help you discover the origins and function of self-harm, to express the feelings that lead to it, and to find other ways of coping with these emotions.

(For further discussion of treatment interventions, mental health professionals should see Chapter 11: Working Toward Change: Therapeutic Techniques to Help Clients Manage Their Feelings and Memories.)

EXPLAINING DISSOCIATION AND CHANGES IN CONSCIOUSNESS

Mental health professionals should help clients to understand and depathologize their dissociative responses. This is done by explaining that dissociation protects abuse survivors from feeling the full intensity of the fear and shock that overwhelmed them at the time of the original traumatic experience. However, while dissociation helps people to survive traumatic experiences, is not adaptive in everyday life after these experiences are over.

Many clients find that information about dissociation and how it functions offers a sense of relief and mastery.

Explain to clients that:

▶   Dissociation is the ability to change consciousness by separating or disconnecting different aspects of awareness. For example, behaviour can be separated from knowledge, as in when a survivor has to sleep with a light on, but has no idea why. Sensations can also be separated from knowledge, as in the example of a trauma survivor who feels nauseated whenever she smells alcohol on someone's breath, but she doesn't know why.

Like intrusive thoughts, memories or ruminations, dissociative responses can be automatically triggered by reminders in the environment. Dissociation reflects the ability to "forget" in order to "survive." Some events are too horrific to be allowed into your consciousness, so your mind has pushed them away and split them off from conscious awareness. Later, these thoughts and feelings may return in the form of intrusive memories and feelings (Allen, 1995).

Dissociation is on a continuum ranging from the experience of:
• getting lost in a daydream,

- driving along the highway and realizing many minutes have gone by while we were in trance-like-state,
- losing time, to
- developing separate parts of oneself (dissociative identities) (Saakvitne et al., 2000).

Dissociation is experienced differently by different people. For some, the experience is like being in a fog, a trance, spacing out or one of complete numbness.

The ability to dissociate usually develops in infancy or childhood as a way of protecting ourselves (an adaptive self-protection). However, this adaptation is limited. Dissociation can create further problems, such as when it becomes an automatic response to feelings that are overwhelming or frightening. This is a problem when a person needs to be taking action to protect herself but instead freezes in a dissociative state.

With practice, people can learn to control dissociation. This is important to learn because dissociation can happen automatically when a trauma survivor feels stressed or emotional pain. Such dissociation can interfere with:
- learning better ways to handle and manage stress and trauma responses
- the ability to remain attentive and focused in therapy and remember what was said and done in sessions
- developing self-protective measures with possible offenders or others who may abuse the trauma survivor.

An example of how dissociation can increase women's vulnerability to revictimization is explained in the following case study. If relevant, it may be useful to share this case study with clients.

CASE STUDY: INCREASED VULNERABILITY TO REVICTIMIZATION

A woman who was sexually abused by her father as a child finds that, as an adult, she becomes panicky and freezes whenever a man talks to her quietly or moves too close to her. She also finds it difficult to remain emotionally and physically present with intimate partners when, in their presence, she is reminded of an action, smell, sound or feeling that she associates with her perpetrator.

In this state of panic, she is unable to appraise the situation to determine how best to respond, or whether she indeed needs to respond to protect herself.

Having been conditioned to respond with an automatic fight-or-flight response, she reacts the same way, whether it is a male stranger or an intimate male partner. When she panics and freezes with a male stranger or acquaintance who is intrusive, she becomes vulnerable to being revictimized.

EXPLAINING CHANGES IN SELF-PERCEPTION

Trauma survivors often perceive themselves as being helpless, ineffectual, stigmatized, and unwanted by others. This perception should gradually transform as the result of the following therapeutic processes.

Explain to clients that:

▶ As you begin to develop skills and tools to negotiate and manage your traumatic stress responses, you will feel a greater sense of self-efficacy and control.

Through developing a secure attachment with the therapist, you will start to experience yourself as respected and valued.

Through psychoeducational approaches that destigmatize and depathologize your adaptations to abuse and neglect, you will feel less isolation and shame.

EXPLAINING DISTURBANCES IN RELATIONSHIPS

Disturbances in relationships is a dimension of complex PTSR that is addressed more in second stage trauma treatment. However, some helpful psychoeducational work can be done in first stage trauma treatment by examining trauma-related beliefs about interpersonal relationships. These beliefs or core relational schemas are often distorted by abuse-related experiences. The schemas that are typically disrupted relate to five central dimensions of:

• intrapersonal experience

- safety
- trust
- esteem
- intimacy and control (Pearlman, 2001).

Distorted schemas can be identified by clients' reports of interpersonal diffi-culties ("I can't trust even my closest friends"), from reports of past events and past conflicts in relationships, and from transference issues that arise with the therapist.

IN GENERAL, WORK ON COGNITIVE SCHEMAS REQUIRES:

- identifying what dimension the distorted schemas relate to (e.g., issues of control and esteem)
- exploring how the distorted schema affects current functioning
- exploring the self-protective value of the distorted schema
- gently challenging the distorted schemas by offering alternative interpretations
- arranging small contained experiments to challenge the distorted schemas or beliefs.

(adapted from Pearlman, 2001)

Some examples of key relational schemas that trauma survivors develop are (from Young, 1999):

- Defectiveness / Shame — "I'm don't want anyone to know me."
- Abandonment / Instability — "People I love will leave me, it's only a matter of time."
- Vulnerability to Harm — "The world is not a safe place."
- Emotional Deprivation — "I never feel close to anyone"
- Subjugation / Self-Sacrifice —"Other people's needs matter more than mine."

It is especially important to explore the dimensions of trust, intimacy and control, safety and esteem with women when addressing the issue of vul-nerability to revictimization.

Many chronically abused women have no template for what healthy rela-tionships are like. Whereas many women would be self-protective if a partner were demeaning or intrusive, abuse survivors will often continue to pursue relationships with men who upset and hurt them. Because many trauma survivors have a limited sense of self, and have not had healthy, mutual relationships, developing and maintaining relationships and maintaining safety from abuse is an ongoing process.

Additionally, the propensity of trauma survivors to dissociate from their bodies when frightened or overwhelmed constricts their capacity to enter into relationships and really know themselves.

Therefore, the work of first stage trauma treatment with women needs to focus on helping survivors contain and manage trauma responses, understand triggers, develop **mindfulness** and connect to their bodies. These tasks are the first order of work before survivors can do the deeper work on establishing relationships.

EXPLAINING SOMATIZATION

Chronic anxiety and emotional numbing get in the way of learning to identify and express one's internal states and wishes. Many abuse survivors suffer from alexithymia, an inability to recognize or describe their feelings. Some experience their feelings only as somatic (bodily) sensations instead of basic emotions, such as anger, joy or fear. This inability to translate somatic states into words causes them to experience emotions as if they were simply physical disturbances or illnesses, rather than psychological states.

Explaining somatization to clients
When outlining the ways in which trauma can be registered in the body, therapists can convey the following type of information to clients.

Explain to clients that:

▶ **Body memory (somatic memory) can hold images, sensations and impulses that are disconnected from conscious knowing. That is to say that your body can "remember" a trauma that your conscious mind is not remembering.**

When the memories of trauma are stored as sensation, similar sensations that you have today can trigger the memories in your body without you being able to make sense of what is happening to you. You experience this as having pain or symptoms in some part of

your body that is somehow connected to trauma, but you don't know what exactly happened.

An important part of healing will be to learn to regulate and contain disturbing sensations.

Intrusive stress responses can be triggered very quickly. The goal of managing intrusive trauma responses is to learn skills that will help you notice when these experiences are coming and to reduce their intensity. You need to be able to stay present with your body, so that you can learn to feel your bodily sensations without needing to dissociate from them.

You also need a good medical doctor who has taken a full history of your experiences and understands the effects of abuse on the body.

Therapists should encourage clients to have any physical problems checked by a doctor.

EXPLAINING ALTERATIONS IN SYSTEMS OF MEANING

A loss of meaning, or sense of purpose, is an aspect of complex post-traumatic stress that should be articulated to clients in first stage trauma treatment.

Explain to clients that:

► It is understandable that people who have experienced severe abuse and neglect no longer believe that life makes sense or has a purpose.

To find meaning and purpose in life again is not part of early stage healing. There is no one road to meaning and purpose but it is helpful to reflect on these questions:
• Why did you survive? For what purpose?
• What helped you keep going?
• What is it that makes your life worth living?
• What advice would you give to someone else who experienced some of the things you have?

CHAPTER 11
Working Toward Change: Therapeutic Techniques to Help Clients Manage Their Feelings and Memories

This chapter begins by outlining the importance of developing a collaborative framework and approach to symptom management. It offers some concrete strategies and tools for treatment, including:

• collaborating with clients to manage symptoms
• an approach for intervening in trauma responses
• steps in symptom management
• developing a tool box.

CHAPTER 11
Working Toward Change: Therapeutic Techniques to Help Clients Manage Their Feelings and Memories

The lives of many abuse survivors are complicated and even controlled by intrusive and persistent responses to trauma. Teaching clients to manage these responses requires knowledge and familiarity with diverse therapeutic tools and strategies. Indeed, this is part of our professional responsibility to clients and to ourselves in embarking on this challenging work.

Mental health professionals working with clients who have frequent and intense responses put a lot of pressure on themselves to try to make them stop. It is easy to feel responsible and anxious when clients are in distress and are asking the therapist to do something to help them.

> Do not lose touch of the central therapeutic goal: giving clients the tools and knowledge they need to feel empowered and to learn skills to manage their own trauma responses.

Therapists need to offer clients a clear, theoretical understanding of any specific approach or technique they are using in trauma work (for example, the information in the first part of the guidebook). Clients gain immense relief from understanding the context and purpose of clinical techniques in therapy. They are also more likely to be willing and able to collaborate with the therapist on managing their trauma responses.

Additionally, not all of these techniques and exercises will be necessary or suited to every client. Not all clients have difficulties in all of the six dimensions of complex post-traumatic stress, nor do all clients struggle with the constellation of responses that constitute simple post-traumatic stress.

Many of the techniques and strategies described are often applicable to a variety of trauma responses, so there will be some overlap. However, the techniques are fully described only once. When they can be applied to other trauma responses, a cross-reference is provided.

COLLABORATING WITH CLIENTS TO MANAGE TRAUMA RESPONSES

The therapeutic relationship is key to the healing process. Working collaboratively with clients to define the problem, and to develop a plan or intervention, recognizes that clients — not therapists — have the ultimate control over their own actions and healing.

Therapists need to determine, with clients, which responses are the most painful and debilitating. They can then work further with clients to rank the responses from most problematic to least. In doing this work, therapists should continue to reframe symptoms as adaptations and to explain the original function of the adaptations. This is a critical part of the ongoing work of normalizing and destigmatizing that helps to attenuate the shame the client might feel.

- Remember that every "symptom" or crisis is the client's attempted solution to a problem.
- Ask what problem the "symptom" is solving and how.
- Attend to the client's ability to manage feelings and traumatic memories.

(adapted from Saakvitne et al., 2000)

Clients will benefit from being taught a systematic approach or framework to intervene in their trauma responses. This approach provides the groundwork for more advanced tools that clients may be taught to manage the current maladaptive nature of trauma responses and to develop more effective coping skills.

AN APPROACH FOR INTERVENING IN
TRAUMA RESPONSES

*Step 1: Recognize, whenever possible, the connection between past experiences and present situations.

▶ In other words, identify triggers and understand the connections. To understand how the past is influencing the present:
   • Assume that your actions make sense in relation to past events.
   • Ask yourself how this behaviour helps you cope.
   • Ask yourself what the behaviour helps you cope with.
   • Ask yourself how your actions are related to your past. Are your current feelings familiar to you? When did you feel this way in childhood?
   • Ask yourself if this is a behaviour you used in the past. Do you understand how it made sense then?
   • Ask yourself if this behaviour is as effective now.
   • Do you have other choices now? What could they be?

Step 2: Separate the past from the present.
Ask the client:

▶ • What in the present reminds you of the past? How does the present feel like the past?
   • Next, list everything in the present that is different from the past.
   • Practise grounding techniques to focus on the present and to bring your body and mind into the present tense, the here and now.
   • Say aloud, "This is now, not then." "It is (year), I am ___ years old." Tell yourself where you are, who you are with.
   • Remind yourself that you have choices now.
   • Remind yourself of resources (like the ability to ask questions, to understand, to leave situations) that you have now that you didn't have then.

*(Saakvitne et al., adapted with permission from The Sidran Press. Copyright 2000.)

Step 3: Exercise control and choice.

▶ • Remind yourself that you have choice because you are an adult now.
   • Think about the consequences of your actions.
   • Choose to slightly alter a coping strategy that you recognize is maladaptive.
   • Make a list of people and services to call.
   • Choose to call someone before you take action alone.
   • Wait for a period of time (e.g., five minutes, one hour) before acting on your impulse. Decide on some activities (e.g., reading) that will distract/delay you from acting impulsively.

EXAMPLE: INTERVENTIONS FOR SYMPTOM MANAGEMENT
Let's make a list of the problems you are having, beginning with the most problematic to the least.

Problem 1: Client feels constant agitation and arousal. Can't stop shakiness.

Problem 2: Client avoids sleeping in her own bed. Stays up late participating in Internet discussion group. Exhausted the next day.

Let's now look at the possible adaptive function of those responses or behaviours.

Problem 1
Client recently had carpets removed from the floor. At bedtime, she heard the floor squeak. Realizes she is shaky and aroused so that she can stay alert to hear if anyone enters her room at night. Remembers in childhood hearing her perpetrator make the floorboards creak when he entered her room.

Adaptive Function: Self-protection

Therapeutic Strategies for Problem 1 — Separate the past from the present.

Client makes a list of the resources she now has as an adult that she didn't have as a child. Realizes that remaining hypervigilant was a childhood self-protection and is not necessary now. Grounds herself by turning the light on in bedroom and focusing on her adult furniture and clothing.

She uses a (mental) container (See "Developing a Container," p. 158) to put away the excess arousal and associated cognitions that were triggered.

Problem 2

Client doesn't want to go bed because she feels afraid that her husband will initiate sexual contact and she will have a flashback.

Adaptive function: Avoidance of painful memories and feelings.

Therapeutic Strategies for Problem 2 — Again, separate the past from the present.

Client recognizes that she is experiencing herself as powerless. Believes that if her husband wants sex, she will have to comply. Accommodating unwanted sex triggers what it felt like when she was sexually abused as a child.

She connects to her body by practising mindfulness and writing her thoughts and feelings in a journal. She is able to recognize that she wants to have physical affection with her husband but not sexual inter-course. She practises establishing boundaries by letting her husband know that she needs him to be physically close to her and hold her but she does not want to be sexual.

THREE STEPS IN MANAGING TRAUMA RESPONSES

There are three major therapeutic steps in managing and reducing trauma effects ("symptoms").

THESE ARE:

1. understanding the problem (recognizing that many "symptoms" are actually coping strategies that are no longer effective)
2. collaboratively developing (with the client) a plan to manage trauma responses
3. working to prevent crises by helping the client develop skills to man-age feelings and traumatic memories.

(Saakvitne et al., 2000)

DEVELOPING A TOOL BOX

> The purpose of skill development is to be better equipped to teach control and management of trauma responses so that clients experience enhanced self-mastery, volition and freedom of choice.
>
> (Chu,1998, p. 268)

The skill development phase of symptom management involves encouraging clients to develop an imaginary set of tools — or "tool box" — to help them manage their trauma responses. In the imaginary tool box, clients can put tools they learn through therapy, as well as tools and resources they create for themselves.

The client tools that will be addressed are:
• trigger awareness
• self-monitoring
• **grounding** techniques
• developing a container
• developing a safe place
• cognitive restructuring
• soothing techniques — imagery and visualizations
• dual awareness
• body awareness and boundary exercises.

Generally there is much overlap in the tools section of this guidebook and the interventions to manage trauma responses (e.g., trigger awareness and grounding for managing dissociative symptoms, flashbacks and self-injurious behaviours). Despite this overlap, the tools will be presented separately in relation to both simple and complex post-traumatic stress responses.

AS OUTLINED IN THE INTRODUCTION, THE SIX CRITERIA FOR DIAGNOSING SIMPLE PTSD INCLUDE:

A. experiencing an event in which the life, physical safety or physical integrity of the client was threatened or actually harmed, resulting in feelings of intense fear, helplessness or horror

B. continuing to re-experience the traumatic event after it is over

C. seeking to avoid reminders of the event

D. exhibiting signs of persistent arousal

E. symptoms last more than one month

F. disturbance causes significant distress in important areas of functioning.

(Reprinted with permission from the *Diagnostic and Statistical Manual of Mental Disorders*, Fourth Edition. Copyright 1994 American Psychiatric Association.)

The remainder of this chapter presents tools to deal with criteria B, C and D.

Criterion B: Re-experiencing

This section presents clinical tools to use for re-experiencing or intrusive reactions (the second criterion of PTSD). The responses to be managed are nightmares, dreams, flashbacks, dissociation and memories.

Containment strategies

Containment strategies are the skills that first need to be developed to control intrusive memories and sensations.

(See "Containment Skill," page 158, for a complete discussion of the application of containment.)

How to help clients with dissociation and flashbacks

Grounding is the most important therapeutic approach for dealing with any form of dissociation or flashback.

THE GOAL OF ANY GROUNDING TECHNIQUE IS TO HELP:

• reconnect the person to the present

• orient the person to the here and now

• connect her to her body and personal control and

• connect her to the therapist and the safe context of the therapy room.

When a client dissociates (which is what happens when a flashback "takes over" and the past becomes the present), therapists can reorient the client by guiding her back to the present situation with their voice. Remember, this technique or intervention is established with the client before actually using it to ground her. The therapist speaks slowly and calmly. Avoid whispering; many perpetrators may have whispered to the client during the original abuse.

Directed awareness (Rothschild, 2000).
Our five senses anchor us in our bodies and surroundings. Clients can reconnect by shifting their awareness from their internal (past) focus to aspects of the external (present) setting. This strategy should be developed collaboratively with the client, using her own words.

Say to clients:

► **Use your visual senses by looking around the room. Name what you see.**

Auditory clues are helpful. You can say to the client:

► **Listen to my voice. I am _____, your therapist. You are in my office. Can you hear my voice? Nod your head if you can hear my voice.**

Together with the client, have a "grounding brainstorm" — brainstorm together to develop ideas for grounding. With clients who often have trouble with flashbacks or dissociation, it is helpful to anticipate this and to suggest making a list of helpful techniques.

Grounding skills
Grounding skills are interventions that help keep a person in the present. These skills usually occur within two specific areas:
1. sensory awareness
2. cognitive awareness.

The following exercises can help clients with grounding skills.

Sensory awareness grounding skills

Spritz your face (with eyes closed), neck, arms and hands with a fine water mister.

Put your feet firmly on the ground.

Listen to soothing music or familiar music you can sing along to. Dance to it. How does it make your body feel?

Rub your palms; clap your hands. Listen to the sound. Feel the sensation.

Hold something that you find comforting. It may be a stuffed animal, a blanket or a favourite sweater. Notice how it feels in your hands. Is it hard or soft?

Carry something meaningful and tangible in your pocket that reminds you of the present. Touch it to remind yourself that you are an adult.

Try to notice where you are and your surroundings, including the people present.

If you have a pet, touch its fur and speak its name out loud.

Exercise. Ride a bike, stationary or otherwise. Lift weights. Do jumping jacks.

▷

Cognitive grounding skills

Reorient yourself in place and time by asking yourself some or all of these questions:

- Where am I?
- What is today?
- What is the date?
- How old am I?
- What season is it?
- Who is the country's political leader?
- What is happening now; what is the context?

The following are examples of behaviours to use for reorientation to place and time:

- Pick up a newspaper or pull up the daily newspaper on your browser. Notice the date and read a current article.

- Call a friend and ask the person to talk with you about something you have done together recently.

- Step outside and determine the temperature. Is it warm? Is the sun shining? Is there a cold breeze? What season is it?

Create a grounding techniques resource list
Therapists can write down grounding techniques that they find useful and would feel comfortable suggesting to a client. Have the client develop a list of grounding techniques, making a large copy for the wall at home and a small copy for her wallet.

Other strategies to strengthen a client's sense of control and choice
Dolan (1991) suggests that the therapist use the following probes to strengthen the client's coping abilities:

▶ • How did you get past those feelings/flashbacks the last time you had them?
- What would be the first small sign that you were calming down? That you were able to handle the flashbacks?
- What do you think the next small sign might be, or has it already happened?
- What did you learn that could help you if you ever felt (or experienced) the feeling/flashback again?

Managing trigger events
Another approach to help clients experience more control is to plan ahead and find ways to deal with triggers before they occur and result in a flashback. Clients need to be reminded that it is important to control their own inner experiences rather than try to avoid everything that triggers their automatic responses.

Some ways to manage triggers include:
- developing a list of triggers that lead to flashbacks or to the unpleasant feelings associated with trauma
- doing relaxation exercises
- doing breathing exercises
- distracting or grounding
- using appropriate medication
- establishing contact with supportive others.

Criterion C: Avoidance and numbing

Ways to reduce numbing
Lessen clients' efforts to try to avoid memories of the trauma. Teach them some titration techniques. (see "Interventions to Help Clients Modulate Their Feelings," page 160).

Encourage them to increase their contact with others, perhaps by joining some type of social organization.

Have them work on triggers that cause them to numb out.

Help them learn to appraise threat by using cognitive techniques (see "Common Beliefs Exercise," page 177).

Encourage them to stay more present in their safe place.

Have them use grounding techniques to separate past trauma from the present.

Criterion D: Hyperarousal and hypervigilance

Ways to reduce arousal
• containment strategies (see "Developing a Container," page 158).
• relaxation techniques
• safe place visualization
• developing dual awareness
• mastery of the fear of arousal (exposure to sensations)
Rather than avoiding symptoms of arousal, the goal is to teach clients how to master the fear of arousal. When clients master the fear of symptoms, anticipatory fear and general arousal will also decrease.

Conduct the following exercise with clients.

Safe place visualization

Clients should be guided to create a safe place in their imagination. This visualization is a skill that, once mastered, can help them whenever they feel overwhelmed.

Conduct the following exercise with clients:

1. Select an image that evokes calm and safety (not the safe place yet — just some image that makes you feel safe and calm).

2. Focus on the image. Feel the emotions. Identify the location of the pleasant sensation in your body. Just allow yourself to experience and enjoy the sensation.

(Therapist allows time for the client to feel the soothing emotions and sensation.)

Where in your body do you feel the sensations?

3. Now bring up the image of your safe place, the place that feels safe and calm to be in. Your safe place can be real or imagined, outdoors or indoors. Maybe you have really been there or maybe you've made it up. You may go there alone, or some person who makes you feel safe can be there. You are in control of it. If you can't think of a safe place, then imagine the safest place you can think of.

4. Notice all your physical senses in that safe place. Notice where you feel the pleasant sensations in your body, and allow yourself to enjoy them. Now concentrate on those sensations.

5. What single word best fits that picture (you can select a word like relax, beach, mountain, etc.)? Think of that word and scene, allowing yourself to again experience the pleasant sensations and a sense of emotional security.

6. Repeat the procedure on your own, bringing up the image and the word and experience the positive emotions and physical sensations.

7. You can use this technique to relax during stressful times. To see how it works, bring up a minor annoyance and notice the accompanying negative feelings. Now use your cueing word, and bring up the emotions and physical sensation of peace and safety. This is called self-cueing with a disturbance.

8. Bring up a disturbing thought once again and access your safe place on your own.

9. Practise this at least once daily. Call up the positive feelings, word, and image while you use the relaxation techniques that you like best.

Developing dual awareness
To manage overwhelming feelings of arousal and panic, clients need to first recognize and accept that the traumatic experience is not occurring in the present time. This can be achieved by developing dual awareness.

Dual awareness is the process of being able to be aware of one or more areas of experience simultaneously. This can be thought of as having one foot in the present, while the other foot is in the past. The focus on dual awareness is to develop a tool in therapy for pacing and containing overwhelming feelings, thoughts or sensations.

Rothschild (2000) explains that survivors have become habituated to paying enormous attention to internal stimuli and misinterpreting them as being associated with past events. She explains that the reconciliation between what we experience in the body and what we perceive outside of the body is lost. For example, when a sensation has been associated with the experience of danger, the perception of any kind of similar sensation may result in the conclusion that danger is imminent in the environment. The perceptual split between internal and external sensory stimuli is referred to as the "experiencing self" and the "observing self" (van der Kolk, 1996).

Developing dual awareness enables the client to address a past traumatic event while secure in the knowledge that the actual present life is safe. The following exercise can help clients develop dual awareness.

Developing dual awareness exercise

Remember a recent mildly distressing event — something that made you feel slightly anxious.

As you remember the event, what do you notice in your body? What happens in your muscles? What happens in your stomach? How does your breathing change? Does your heart rate increase or decrease? Do you become warmer or colder? If there is any change in temperature, is it everywhere in your body or is it focused in one place?

Now bring your awareness back into the room where you are. Notice the colour of the walls, the texture of the carpet. What is the temperature of this room? What do you smell here? Does your breathing change as your focus of awareness changes?

Now try to keep this awareness of your present surroundings while you remember the slightly distressing event. Is it possible for you to maintain awareness of where you are physically as you remember that event?

End this exercise by refocusing your awareness on your current surroundings.

Further ways of managing arousal and anxiety

Further ways of managing arousal and anxiety include helping the client with the following:

- Face the trauma responses. Confront them until they no longer matter. The body is able to adapt to the stress response. The mind becomes sharper under stress.
- Willingly accept the symptoms. Relax, let go, and invite in the body's responses. Realize that, with time, the arousal and the intensity of the symptoms will diminish.
- Float. With a deeply relaxed body, breathe gently and peacefully and see yourself floating forward as if in a cloud or on the water. There is no struggle or clenching of muscles; these increase arousal. Likewise, trying to forget memories also creates tension.
- Let time pass. A sensitized nervous system will not be soothed overnight. Allow time for your body to readjust its chemical balance and to learn new ways to react to stressors (from Weekes, 1984).

Ask the client:

▶   "How strong were those feelings of anxiety and arousal, on a scale of one to 100?"

CLIENTS SHOULD BE TAUGHT TO OBSERVE AND DESCRIBE:
- events that prompt emotions
- their interpretation of these events, their physical sensations
- their behaviours that express emotions.

Emotional regulation is enhanced by increasing positive experiences. Clients are taught to increase short-term positive experiences and decrease painful ones.

CHAPTER 12
Strategies and Tools for Managing Complex Post-Traumatic Stress Responses

This chapter offers strategies and tools for managing responses from the following four dimensions of complex post-traumatic stress:
• affect dysregulation
• dissociation and changes in consciousness
• changes in self-perception
• somatization.

It includes therapeutic approaches in:
• affect and emotional regulation strategies and self-soothing skills
• reducing anxiety through visualization
• identifying and labelling emotions
• assigning meaning to events
• grounding
• treatment strategies for self-harming behaviours
• strategies for dealing with dissociation and traumatic amnesia
• body awareness and developing anchors
• treatment strategies for working with changes in self-perception
• addressing cognitive schemas that maintain trauma responses.

CHAPTER 12
Strategies and Tools for Managing Complex Post-Traumatic Stress Responses

First stage trauma treatment primarily addresses the following four dimensions:
1. (dimension one) affect dysregulation
2. (dimension two) dissociation and changes in consciousness
3. (dimension three) changes in self-perception
4. (dimension five) somatization.

These dimensions will be presented with the techniques and tools that help trauma clients bring their trauma responses under control.

Clients can gradually achieve control over intrusive responses, but only if the client and therapist work together to manage and control the rate and nature of re-experiencing past abuse. Education about how this can be done is the most important intervention in pacing this stage of the therapy. Mental health professionals must feel confident and skilled in their use of these techniques. Unless therapists truly believe that the responses associated with severe post-traumatic stress — affect dysregulation and dissociative disorders — can be modulated and controlled, they will be unable to convince clients of this.

Chu (1998) explains that clients struggle with this proposition because they consider their responses to be out of their control. He explains that efforts made to control re-experiencing responses are at odds with the client's own internal experience that control is impossible to achieve.

> Helplessness is at the core of trauma, and it erodes the development and experience of self-efficacy. Control, on the other hand, is the antidote to helplessness. The process of achieving adequate control is difficult and gradual. Early attempts may be only minimally successful.

Chu emphasizes that it is essential to achieve control over re-experiencing responses; without repeated effort, this goal will not be reached, and the client will not achieve some stability in her life.

DIMENSION ONE: AFFECT REGULATION STRATEGIES
Affect regulation strategies include developing the tools and resources necessary to recognize, observe, modulate and cope with affects that a client experiences. In developing these skills and tools, clients are better able to cope with disturbing affects as they arise.

> **THE KEY STRATEGIES AND SKILLS REQUIRED FOR AFFECT REGULATION ARE:**
> - containment
> - modulation
> - identifying feelings
> - mindfulness
> - addressing self-harming behaviours.

Containment skill
Affect regulation begins with developing containment strategies. This is considered the first skill that needs to be developed, because it effectively controls the intrusive trauma memories, schemas, images and disturbing physiological sensations that overwhelm trauma survivors. These overwhelming feelings or thoughts often lead to harmful behaviour and make it extremely difficult for clients to focus on their therapy. Learning effective containment skills empowers and reassures the client.

Developing a container
Instructions to the client:

▶ Many people who have experienced personal trauma can often become overwhelmed by disturbing feelings or thoughts. Learning to develop and to use containment images and techniques can give you a sense of calm and control over these disturbing feelings.

Containment is a tool that allows you to put away disturbing thoughts, images, feelings and body sensations for exploration later.

The strategy of containment does not mean that you are losing part of yourself or that you are denying your feelings and experiences. Creating a container gives you much-needed relief from recurrent, intrusive thoughts and feelings that can retraumatize you.

When you learn additional skills to manage your feelings, you can then decide to examine some of these thoughts and feelings by removing them from your container one at a time or in small amounts.

Note: Some clients will insist they do not have the capacity or skill to contain symptoms and that this is a crazy idea. If this happens, therapists can explain that we all have the ability to dissociate or avoid painful material. Most trauma survivors do dissociate or have done so in the past. It helps to explain that containing is making the conscious choice to dissociate painful material, and that dissociation is a mechanism they already have but will now be able to develop more control over.

Following this introduction to the concept of containment, ask the client to design and visualize a container that is strong enough to hold her disturbing thoughts, feelings, sensations and images. Have the client take the time to carefully visualize the container, so she has a clear image of it and has considered its form, location and function. Explain that the container has a special slot, similar to a bank deposit, that allows her to add any new material to the container without any disturbing material escaping.

Some clients benefit from the idea of a notice on the container that states: "To be opened only when it helps me in my healing."

Some of the containers that clients can create include:
- a steel vault, chained and welded, buried under the ground or in the sea, to confine flashbacks
- glass jars or Rubbermaid containers containing grief, sadness or other emotions
- a video cassette stored in a cupboard for later viewing of traumatic events
- computer discs with information related to the traumatic experiences or events.

159

The type of container the client develops will provide information about her subjective appraisal of the magnitude of their disturbing material. In some cases an inadequately conceptualized container, a "flimsy shoe box" for example, shows that a client is not feeling safe with the process or is ill-prepared to do the exercise.

Once the container is well visualized and conceptualized, the therapist then has the client identify one intrusive thought, overwhelming feeling, or disturbing bodily sensation that she would like to contain. This can be done by asking the client to first do a body scan and then locate the sensation and where it is held. Ask the client what percentage of the disturbing sensations, feelings or thoughts she wishes to contain. When that is determined, have the client visualize putting every disturbing thing into her container and then sealing it shut.

Other emotional regulation skills (modulation)

Interventions to help clients modulate their feelings
Therapists can suggest several techniques to help clients decrease the frequency and intensity of their upsetting internal states, and to give them a greater sense of self-efficacy and mastery. It is important to emphasize that the goal is not necessarily to eradicate their trauma responses, but to increase their control of them.

> Visualization techniques are often useful to clients, especially when the techniques contain suggestions of how to change the intensity of a feeling. Clients can use visualization techniques to help soothe themselves, feel less anxious and experience things less intensely.

It helps to explain that modulating emotions is similar to using a regulator. Regulators are used to turn things both up and down. Clients need to understand that they can increase and decrease the intensity of feelings. They can turn painful feelings down or turn pleasant feelings up. They may need different regulators to manage different problems, such as:
• numb or disconnected feelings
• intrusive images
• racing thoughts.

Images commonly used to regulate thoughts, feelings and impulses include a:
• car brake
• dimmer switch
• remote control
• faucet
• thermostat.

The following exercise can help clients regulate their feelings.

Increasing control over your feelings

Dimmer switch

Visualize a dial with numbers on it from 0 to 10. A number controls the intensity of whatever feeling you are having. Perhaps you are feeling sad. Imagine turning the dial toward 0 and turning down the intensity of your sadness, just as you could dim the intensity of light with a dimmer switch. A dimmer switch lessens the amount of electrical energy that can be emitted. Imagine you have the capacity to lessen the amount of energy that is expressed in your sadness. Allow yourself to slowly and gradually diminish the feeling.

Remote control

This device can be used to control the intensity of intrusive images or sounds. Imagine changing channels, switching from disturbing images to soothing images. You may want to develop a "safe place" channel and run an imaginary video of the safe place you created. You can use your remote to decrease the volume of sounds or voices you hear in your head or fast forward though a flashback.

Riding a train

Imagine you are on a comfortable seat in a train, going on a journey. You are sitting back, looking out the window at the landscape. The landscape is made up of your emotional feelings. You can watch your feelings pass by as you sit comfortably in your seat. You can look out with curiosity and bring feelings closer to you. You can make them small and distant like a speck on the horizon. Or you can choose to close your eyes and just feel the comfortable motion of the train on the tracks, knowing that you are in motion and that your feelings too will pass by, just like the scenery out the window.

Split screen

This skill is like watching a television screen where two consecutive programs are playing. Divide a mental TV screen, putting the past on one side and the present on the other. You have the remote control that allows you to mute, slow down, fast forward, pause, turn to black and white, or turn off the program completely. You can download the disturbing memories to a videotape for three seconds. You can then turn off the TV, take out the tape and store or file it in a safe place.

▷

The videotape (especially helpful with memories)

Your feeling is on this videotape. You have the remote control in your hand. At any time, you can turn it on or off, change the volume, pause it, fast forward or rewind it, hit the mute button or take the tape out and pack it away in a secure place.

The audio tape

Visualize a cassette tape player. Your emotion is on the cassette. You can shut it off. You can turn the volume down so you can't hear it. Turn it up a tiny bit, so you can barely hear it. Turn it up another bit, so it is very soft. Turn it down again. Practise until you are ready to turn it up just enough to hear it. Remember, you can turn it off or down whenever you want.

Other visualization techniques can be used to help clients feel both grounded and connected to their bodies. The following images can be called up in conjunction with guided relaxation techniques.

Self-soothing

Light stream technique
Ask the client to concentrate on the upsetting body sensations. Identify the following by asking the questions:

▶ 1. If the upsetting body sensation had a _____

    a) shape   d) temperature
    b) size   e) texture
    c) colour   f) sound (high pitched or low)

    what would it be?

2. What is the colour you associate with healing?

3. Imagine that a light in this colour is coming in through the top of your head and directing itself at the shape in your body. Let's pretend that the source of this light is the cosmos so the more you use, the more you have available. <u>The light directs itself at the shape and penetrates, permeates, resonates and vibrates in and around it.</u> As it does, what happens to the shape?

If the client says that it is changing in any way, continue repeating the underlined portion and asking for feedback, until the shape/size/colour/etc. is completely gone. Its disappearance usually correlates with the upsetting feeling also dissolving. After she feels better, bring the light into every portion of her body, and give her a positive suggestion for peace and calm until the next session. Ask the client to become alert and aware at the count of five.

Reducing anxiety through visualization
Teach clients the Spiral Technique:

▶ Identify and locate the anxiety feeling(s) in your torso.

Now, in your mind, give it a spiral shape, like a corkscrew.

After you have located the place in your body where anxiety is expressed, and have identified the anxiety with a particular image, notice in what direction the anxiety is spiralling. Reverse the direction.

Takes a deep breath and imagine the spiral unwinding in the opposite direction, slowly, slowly, until it comes to a stop and disappears.

Identifying and labelling emotions

Many clients have spent their lives avoiding their feelings and avoiding connecting to their bodies. As a result, they are not able to differentiate and identify different emotional states. Emotional regulation begins with noticing. Learning to identify and label emotions requires the ability to observe one's own responses and to recognize the context in which the emotion occurs.

The elements that best define this process are:

1 the event prompting the emotion
2. the interpretations of the event that resulted in the emotion
3. the physical sensation of the emotion
4. the behaviours used to express the emotion
5. the after-effects of the emotion on other types of functioning.

Explain to clients:

▶ An important way to increase emotional control is to learn how to identify your automatic thoughts. Usually, our negative emotional responses are directly preceded by automatic thoughts. Usually, we are not trained to recognize these thoughts and are probably not aware of them.

For exercises on automatic thoughts, see "Common Beliefs Exercise," page 177, and "Self Monitoring Chart," page 172.

Assigning meaning to events

Most of our emotions are a result of how we interpret events around us. Many people think that our emotional responses are directly caused by outside events and situations.

▶ For example, a friend does not call you when she said they would. Your response is one of fury and feelings of rejection.

Later, you discover that the friend had a significant emergency arise, which prevented her from calling.

This shifts your interpretation of and reaction to the event. This shows that our emotional response to an external event partly hinges on the meaning we attach to it.

Grounding

Grounding techniques are the methods used to increase mindfulness (see "Mindfulness," page 181).

The purpose of teaching grounding is to help clients increase their awareness in the here and now, to reduce post-traumatic stress responses such as flashbacks, intrusive re-experiencing and dissociation.

Grounding is the process of being present and connected to the here and now. It can be explained to clients that, if they are paying attention to the present, then they are less likely to be lost in the past with no awareness of present-day resources. Present, focused awareness allows for increased coping with, and protection against being trapped in, helpless feelings of the past.

Treatment strategies for self-harming behaviours

These self-harming behaviours might include:
• self-injury
• eating disorders
• substance use problems
• other addictions.

REMEMBER THAT SELF-HARMING BEHAVIOUR SERVES A PURPOSE.
• How does this behaviour help the client?
• What problem does it try to solve?

The function or goals of self-harming behaviours can usually be classified under one of the following categories:

- to manage — by expressing or blocking — strong feelings
- to replace emotional pain with physical pain
- to manage other behaviour
- to create or maintain dissociation
- to interrupt dissociation (to feel real)
- to remember trauma without consciously knowing it
- to enforce internal rules for self-control (e.g., "I don't want anything; don't need anyone; don't have sexual feelings")
- to relieve mounting internal tension
- to communicate distress to others
- to punish the self or others.

Interventions with self-harming behaviours
First, therapists must identify and respect the function of the self-harming behaviour before supporting the survivor's capacity to choose alternative solutions. This is done by exploring and understanding the usefulness of the self-harming behaviour.

Acknowledging the function of self-harming is often a relief to clients, who have expected to be judged and told that they are crazy. Others feel validated to learn that someone can understand their behaviour in a helpful way. Some clients are taught "chain analyses" to help them understand the sequence of the internal and external events that have led to their self-harming behaviour (see "Develop a chain analysis of the sequence of events," p. 173).

Once the function of the behaviour has been respectfully acknowledged, the therapist should then work with clients to develop alternative coping behaviours, and to help clients recognize, understand and talk about the experience of inner tension.

Strategies to address specific functions of self-harm
In relation to the following expressed needs, therapists can suggest the following alternative behaviours to clients.

167

Alternatives to self-harm

Physical awareness/sensation
Hold an ice cube against your skin. Take a shower and rub your skin with a cloth or brush. Put a rubber band on your wrist and snap it a few times. Rub a cool lotion over your skin. Ride a bike fast and far. Carry safe, comforting objects, crystals, smooth stones, etc.

Delaying/distracting
Take a shower. Read a book. Go out and be around people. Dig in your garden. Call a friend. Write in your journal.

Expressing anger through activities
Break something safe. Break old crockery or glass bought at a junk store. Smash ice cubes. Throw eggs in the shower. Rip apart an old phone book. Punch or scream into a pillow.

Non-harmful symbolic enactments
Draw red lines on arms with a felt marker. Draw red lines on paper, then slowly drip water on the ink and watch it spread. Cut a box or a stuffed animal.

Tension reduction
Exercise. Pluck hair on your leg with tweezers. Do yard work. Vacuum the house.

Express your feelings
Draw the feeling. Write a letter to someone you care about. Write in code. Whisper into a pillow. Write what you are feeling. Don't edit; allow a stream of consciousness. Write down the reasons why you believe you need to be punished. Bring your list to your therapist. Remind yourself that you are already being punished by feeling such self-blame.

Create calmness/self-soothing
Create a safe place. Put the disturbing feelings into an imaginary container. Listen to a relaxation tape. Talk to someone supportive. Listen to tapes of a friend or a therapist talking. Have a bubble bath. Listen to music. Create art. Walk outdoors and notice the natural surroundings. Meditate.

DIMENSION TWO: DISSOCIATION AND CHANGES IN CONSCIOUSNESS

Therapists need to explain to clients that their dissociative responses were adaptive at the time that the traumatic events happened to them. It should be emphasized that these responses made it possible for clients to survive.

However, unlike emotional dysregulation, which many clients find intolerable and difficult to deal with, many clients find dissociative responses to be momentarily satisfying and have not critically assessed the limitations of this adaptive response. Therefore, the first task for the therapist is to help increase a client's awareness of the role of dissociation in the client's life and the limitations it has imposed.

The key strategies and skills required for dealing with dissociation include:
• developing a rationale for wanting to modify dissociative responses (understanding that dissociation has helped the person survive and recognizing its limitations now as a coping response)
• recognizing the triggers that lead to dissociation
• practising grounding techniques that can help prevent or modify dissociation cognitive restructuring.

DISSOCIATIVE ADAPTATIONS THAT REDUCE INTERNAL AWARENESS INCLUDE:
1. trance-inducing behaviour/self-hypnosis
2. switching (moving into different personality states)
3. time loss
4. amnesia
5. depersonalization (out-of-body experiences)
6. derealization (feeling in a dream-like state).

Trauma survivors may think they still need these responses to protect themselves. However, they must understand that dissociation can be maladaptive. It is useful to have clients recognize the differences between dissociation and self-awareness. The following exercise by Vermilyea (2000) can help clients develop this initial awareness. Give clients this chart and have them add other differences that they notice for themselves.

The differences between dissociation and self-awareness

Dissociation / Avoidance / Numbing	Self-Awareness
makes you unaware of what's going on inside you	makes you aware of what's going on inside you
makes you feel safe but does not make you safe	increases your safety by making you aware of resources
makes it hard to solve problems	increases your awareness of choices
reduces your self-control	increases your self-control
limits your access to your feelings	gives you access to your feelings
(add your own differences here)	(add your own differences here)
_____	_____
_____	_____
_____	_____
_____	_____
_____	_____
_____	_____
_____	_____
_____	_____
_____	_____
_____	_____
_____	_____
_____	_____

(Vermilyea, E.G. *Growing Beyond Survival: A Self-Help Toolkit for Managing Traumatic Stress.* Reprinted with permission from Sidran Press. Copyright 2000. The full *Growing Beyond Survival* curriculum is available from Sidran Press: www.sidran.org or 410.825.8888.)

Additional approaches to dealing with dissociation

1. Identifying triggers

The first step in this process is to explain the concept of triggers and the different types of triggers (current stressors, stimuli reminiscent of the abuse, smells or certain types of touch, anniversary effects).

For example, the therapist can say to clients:

► Triggers are cues from the outside environment or from your own inside environment (inner life) that tap into childhood feelings. Being triggered is a normal and common consequence of childhood abuse.

Survivors may feel more in control if they can
• anticipate that they will be triggered
• recognize what their triggers are
• develop strategies to ground themselves when they are triggered.

Once a survivor can recognize that she has been triggered, she can choose a course of action.

Explore with clients situations that are likely to trigger flashbacks. The following are probing questions that will help clients identify their triggers:

► • Is there something going on in your life right now that reminds you of how you felt during the traumatic time?
• In what ways are the current and past situation similar?
• What aspects of the experience are most likely to trigger your flashbacks?
• What do theses images, thoughts, feelings or sensations mean to you?

Have clients identify the different types of triggers that they are aware of:
• media coverage of violence
• particular conversations
• certain types of people
• current stressors or losses
• smells or touch
• dates/anniversaries.

Have clients self-monitor by using the following chart:

Self monitoring chart

Trigger	Negative Self-Talk	Emotional / Behavioural Physical Consequence	Coping Strategies
What set this in motion? (internal or external event)	What did you say to yourself?	What did you feel emotionally? What did you do? What did you feel in your body?	What did you do to try to cope?

Trigger:
Self-monitoring includes identifying the trigger, when it happened, where you were, what you were doing and who you were with.

Negative self-talk:
Record what you said to yourself. If you can remember, also include your evaluation or interpretation of the experience.

Consequence:
Note your emotional, behavioural and physical reactions.

Coping strategies:
Record how you coped with the situation.

Alternatively, you could record these observations in a journal.

2. What to do when triggered
When triggered, the first coping strategy survivors can use is to get grounded:
• Remind themselves that that was then and this is now.
• Remember that triggers are about someone else, somewhere else, doing something else.

Following this basic intervention, a number of other techniques may be used either individually or in combination.

Treating dissociative phenomena

Step 1. Analyse behaviour
Behavioural analysis is used to develop a thorough account of the events, cognitions and emotions that precede and follow the dissociative behaviour, to understand the factors that elicit and maintain the behaviour. This step is essential to determine the most effective points and procedures for intervention.

The client gives a precise and detailed description of the dissociative behaviour. Questions that should be asked by the therapist include:

▶   • **Could you describe for me what you experienced?**
    • **How long did that feeling last?**
    • **Did you have any thoughts at the time?**
    • **Did you have any feelings at the time? What were they?**

Step 2. Develop a chain analysis of the sequence of events
Develop a chain analysis of the sequence of events, preceding and following the dissociative episode, to identify possible cues and precipitating events.

Questions for the beginning of the chain analysis include:

▶   • **When did you first start dissociating?**
    • **What set that off?**
    • **What was going on at the moment you started dissociating?**
    • **What did you do while dissociating?**

Step 3. Decrease the availability of cues
Clients can decrease the availability of cues by using such techniques as:
• distracting with other activities

- engaging in activities that elicit opposite emotions
- pushing the situation away by leaving it or blocking thoughts
- engaging in self-soothing activities and skills for improving the moment (imagery, relaxation or taking brief vacations).

Step 4. Regulate emotional responses to traumatic cues
Mindfulness and emotional regulation skills can help clients regulate their emotional responses to traumatic cues.

DIMENSION THREE: CHANGES IN SELF-PERCEPTION

Trauma survivors often struggle with a sense of self that is primarily viewed as worthless, helpless, ineffectual and undesirable to others. Many trauma clients have never been reflected in a positive way in their relationships. Often, the adaptations they developed in response to the abuse (not trusting others, angry outbursts, constant crises, emotional disconnection) result in troubled and difficult relationships. Trauma clients don't often expect that they will be understood by others or that their trauma responses would be respected and understood. As a result, much of the healing work on survivors' perceptions of self will be done through therapeutic attunement.

Despite the core work that needs to happen in a corrective therapeutic relationship, survivors can additionally benefit from tools that help them understand that some of their negative cognitions keep them stuck believing negative ideas about themselves and others. Therefore, cognitive restructuring is an important therapeutic tool.

Second, the greatest antidote to feeling helpless and powerless are experiences of self-efficacy and self-control. Teaching survivors symptom management tools will help them experience themselves more positively.

One other important therapeutic tool used primarily by **Eye Movement Desensitization and Reprocessing** (EMDR) therapy is the idea of positive resource installation, whereby clients recall positive moments in their lives, moments where they felt effective, strong, in control or they felt like a kind, loving person. These experiences are installed and enhanced using EMDR.

Treatment strategies for working with changes in self-perception

> **THE THERAPEUTIC STRATEGIES FOR WORKING WITH CHANGES IN SELF-PERCEPTION INCLUDE:**
> - therapeutic alliance
> - cognitive restructuring
> - positive resource installation (this is not elaborated on in this guide-book, but see Leeds and Shapiro, 2000).
> - global skill development to manage trauma responses (see above exercises).

Addressing cognitive schemas that maintain trauma responses

a) Identifying trauma-related thinking
By reading over a client's self-monitoring chart, therapists often learn that the client believes that she is crazy or helpless, and/or that no one is to be trusted. These cognitive schemas often trigger dissociative episodes and other distressing symptoms.

b) Cognitive processing / restructuring — how to challenge trauma-related thinking
Cognitive restructuring can be used to teach trauma survivors that their beliefs are often associated with negative feelings (anger, fear or guilt). The therapist works with the client to replace distorted or inaccurate thoughts with more adaptive thinking. Of course, if the thoughts or beliefs are accurate, it is important to validate them and help the client develop plans and behaviours to ensure her safety.

Explain to clients that:

▶   Often, when people have suffered a traumatic and emotionally painful event, their thinking is shaped by the experience. Many survivors have told us that their thoughts about themselves and others have become negative as a result of the abuse they have suffered.

Because we know that feelings and behaviours are linked to thoughts and beliefs, it is important to identify any negative trauma-related thoughts that are causing you distress.

175

We will review a list of common cognitive distortions so that you can begin to identify any errors in logic you may be making that lead to unpleasant and distressing thinking and feeling.

The goal of cognitive restructuring is to help you identify negative thoughts, evaluate their accuracy, challenge and discard them or do something to decrease your negative thoughts and feelings.

c) Client worksheets

The following exercise can help clients identify and rate their troublesome beliefs.

Common Beliefs Exercise

Listed below are common beliefs/thoughts held by people who have survived abuse. Please read these thoughts/beliefs and place a check mark to the left of each statement that applies to you. Then rate how much you believe each thought (from 0% to 100%).

If you wish, please add other troublesome beliefs to the list. We will examine the helpfulness and accuracy of these beliefs in future sessions.

Self Thoughts %

I am damaged.

I am not loveable.

I am responsible for what happened to me.

It's my fault.

I am bad.

I am helpless.

I am incompetent.

I should have fought harder.

I shouldn't have frozen.

I should have said "no."

I shouldn't have worn that outfit.

I shouldn't have walked alone at night.

I will never be able to date again.

I am damaged.

I cannot be trusted.

I am going crazy or I am crazy.

I am vulnerable.

I will never be the same again.

Other/World

The world is a dangerous place.

Men cannot be trusted.

Women cannot be trusted.

People cannot be trusted.

I will be raped again.

People are bad.

People are cruel.

People take advantage of me.

No one can help me.

The world is a dangerous place.

People are violent by nature.

There is no good in the world.

There is not safety in the world.

No one cares about me.

People can hurt me.

People can assault me.

Bad things happen everywhere.

The world is a bad place.

(From Diana Hearst-Ikeda, PhD, *CBT Materials for Therapists and Clients*. Reprinted with permission from VA Boston Healthcare System. Copyright © 2000.)

Cognitive restructuring

Client worksheet
According to cognitive theories, negative thoughts are often responsible for depressed and anxious mood and behaviours.

Explain to clients that:

► As a result of the trauma, you have probably come to believe that the world is a bad and dangerous place, and that you are helpless. You may not be able to trust other people, and may believe that you are unable to cope with stress.

You may believe these thoughts 100 per cent, which leads to anxiety, depression, avoidance of situations and people, and feelings of helplessness and hopelessness.

The facts

The world is not 100 per cent safe, nor is it 100 per cent dangerous. Sometimes bad things happen, and sometimes good things happen to people.

Recovering from trauma means that you will need to learn to accurately assess the safety and danger of certain situations, and challenge your negative trauma-related thinking to lead a happy, productive life.

Beginning to challenge your thinking
Part of the therapeutic work of first stage trauma treatment involves teaching clients to become aware of their negative thoughts and associated feelings and behaviours.

Have your clients answer the following questions and do the following:

► *Are my beliefs accurate?*

Consider whether you are using faulty or distorted logic to support the accuracy of your negative beliefs.

Collect evidence or conduct an experiment (e.g., talk to someone if you have been making assumptions) to find out if your belief is accurate.

Ask yourself questions from the Challenging Questions Worksheet to find out what significance this belief has for you.

If your thought is not accurate, you can reject it. There is no point in continuing to believe an inaccurate thought that makes you feel distressed.

However, if it is accurate, we will together need to come up with solutions and behaviours to decrease your anxiety.

Give clients a copy of the Challenging Questions Worksheet (following page).

Challenging questions worksheet

What evidence do I have to support this belief?

What is the evidence to contradict this belief?

Is there another way of looking at this thought/situation?

What would I say to a friend who held the same belief?

Am I using faulty logic or emotional reasoning (reasoning on the basis of feeling versus fact) to support this belief?

Am I making assumptions about what others are thinking or feeling? Is this an example of extreme thinking or catastrophizing?

If this thought is true, so what?

If this thought is true, what can I do about it?

What does it really mean to me or about me now?

What will it mean to me in the future?

What would it mean to give up this belief?

What would my life be like if I gave up this belief?

Are my interpretations of the situation too far removed from reality to be accurate?

Is it helpful for me to think this way about myself? About others?

Am I confusing a feeling with a thought? A thought with a feeling?

Am I taking examples out of context?

Am I confusing a low-probability event with a high-probability event?

(From Diana Hearst-Ikeda, PhD, *CBT Materials for Therapists and Clients*. Reprinted with permission from VA Boston Healthcare System. Copyright © 2000.)

General rules for cognitive challenging

▶ While asking yourself the preceding questions, if you discover that your belief is not accurate, you can throw it out or reject it. What's the sense of holding onto negative, inaccurate beliefs that make you feel badly about yourself and others?

If your belief is accurate, you should probably do something to decrease your negative thinking and associated negative feelings. For example, if you discover that you live in a dangerous neighbourhood, you may wish to move or get a security alarm. There is no reason to convince yourself that you live in a safe place if you do not.

DIMENSION FIVE: SOMATIZATION

Treatment strategies for somatization include:
• cognitive behavioural therapy (CBT) (see page 178)
• relaxation strategies (see page 164)
• EMDR (see page 174)
• body awareness (mindfulness).

Body awareness

Rothschild (2000) explains that body awareness can be developed to become an important therapeutic tool. Body awareness makes it possible to gauge, slow down, and stop hyperarousal, and help separate the past from the present. She emphasizes that body awareness is the first step toward interpreting somatic memory.

Ogden and Minton (2000) explain that mindfulness is the key to becoming more aware of internal sensori-motor responses. Mindfulness is the process of focusing one's awareness in the here-and-now, to simply observe internal experiences rather than try to change the experience.

Mindfulness

Teach mindfulness by asking the following questions:

▶ • What do you feel in your body?
• Where exactly do you experience tension?
• What sensation do you feel in your legs right now?
• What happens in the rest of your body when your hand makes a fist?

Note: When clients are unable to feel their body sensation at all, or they do not have the vocabulary to describe their sensations, the approach is slightly modified:

▶ • **Do a scan of your entire body, starting at the top of your head, through your limbs, torso, and back, hands and feet.**
  • **What sensations are you aware of?**

If they are still not aware of any sensations, ask them to take one hand and squeeze the opposite arm for several seconds:

▶ • **Now, just sit and feel the sensations in the arm that you squeezed.**
  • **What are you aware of feeling?**

(Ogden & Minton, reprinted with permission from Sensorimotor Psychotherapy Institute. Copyright © 2000.)

Basic introduction to recognizing sensations
Many trauma survivors cannot differentiate pleasure and neutral sensations from disturbing ones. As a result, all sensations become threatening, and survivors work to avoid feeling or connecting to them. Mental health professionals can reintroduce clients to the function of sensations by explaining that:

▶ Sensations have an important function. They help us gauge physiological and emotional needs. They tell us when we are tired, in pain, hungry, thirsty, cold, warm, comfortable, happy, excited, worried, etc.

Without being able to feel pain or the sensations that indicate fear, we would be vulnerable to harm.
  • How would you know the bath water was too hot to get into?
  • How would you know not to approach a dog on the street?
  • How would you know not to answer your door to an unknown person late at night?

Contrary to what many therapists believe, clients usually become less anxious, rather than more, when they are encouraged to notice and describe their body sensation under this quick scan method. Once they become adept at it, many clients report that it is a relief for them to shift focus to current sensations. Body awareness can become a secure link to the present.

Body awareness & boundary exercises

1. Skin as a boundary

Rub the surface of your skin (without massaging muscles) with your own hand, a towel, a pillow, or against a wall.

Feel where clothes touch skin, where body meets chair.

Tell yourself, "This is me. This is where I start/stop. This is my boundary."

Distinguish boundaries with another, using safe touch.

2. Solidity of bones

Feel your spine against the wall, sitting, standing.

Tap the bones at your elbow, wrist, knee, ankle.

3. Muscular tension

Tense parts that feel vulnerable or shaky.

Use a hard chair/upright posture.

Feel the muscular resistance in your legs, arms, internally.

Compare stretching and tensing.

4. Language to focus on body sensations

You're feeling unsafe? How do you know?

Where do you feel it in your body?

Do you know that kind of sensation?

What is it like?

What happens in your body when you acknowledge it?

(Rothschild, B. *The Body Remembers: The Psychophysiology of Trauma and Trauma Treatment*. Copyright 2000, W.W. Norton & Company, Inc. Reprinted with permission. To photocopy this exercise, permission must be obtained from W.W. Norton & Company, Inc. 500 Fifth Ave., New York 10110. www.wwnorton.com.)

Developing positive resources

Once a client becomes more connected to her sensations and bodily experiences, she can learn to use body awareness to develop resources to give herself relief and well-being. For example, positive memories in a client's body and mind can be used to develop the idea of a positive resource or anchor.

Positive resources can be drawn from experiences in the client's life, such as a soothing, comforting spot in nature (a garden, or lake), a loved pet, a person who supported her in her life, or an activity that she remembers feeling competent and comforted by (woodworking or gardening).

Once she develops this positive resource or anchor, the therapist should ask her to imagine herself involved with this positive image or activity.

CASE STUDY: DEVELOPING AN ANCHOR OR POSITIVE RESOURCE

One female client described the sense of safety and well-being she felt whenever she took her dog, a great dane named Hero, for a walk. To connect her to these positive sensations, her therapist would ask her to imagine walking through the park with Hero and describe everything she felt in her body. The client would describe the calmness in her chest and stomach, her back and shoulders would relax, and she would feel an incredible strength, power and freedom. Her therapist would then ask her to complete this positive belief about herself, "I am _____." She would respond, "I am strong."

Once this positive resource is developed, it can be applied to moments when the client is feeling powerless, disconnected, hyperaroused, etc. The therapist gave the following directions:

"I want you to remember being with Hero for a few minutes. Imagine that you are walking along the street with him."

The resource can be strengthened by providing sensory cues that the client has described as being part of this anchor.

Rothschild (2000) explains that inserting anchors lowers the base level of hyperarousal that a client is experiencing. By doing this, the therapist paces the therapy, bringing the client into her own strengths and resources by connecting her to her own somatic memories, and teaching emotional regulation.

Conclusion

Working with women whose abuse histories have led them to suffer with complex post-traumatic stress is challenging, complicated, and very important work. It is also highly skilled work, which must be carefully paced. Ultimately, it is also a very rewarding process.

In undertaking this work, mental health professionals must also engage in some self-care, both to retain the energy and focus required to provide excellent care to our clients, and to make the work manageable for ourselves.

One of the ways we need to maintain our own optimism and hopefulness is by being able to recognize small and incremental successes in our clients' lives. Part of the skill of this work, therefore, also lies in being able to impart a sense of hopefulness to our clients. Because knowledge about the effects of trauma is expanding so rapidly, there is a parallel increase in our knowledge about effective ways to offer therapeutic support and relief from traumatic effects to our clients. This means that many women can expect to be helped with appropriate, specialized therapeutic interventions and support. It is hoped the analysis and information in this guidebook will contribute to these efforts.

Resources

Selected Readings on Complex PTSR for Therapists

Courtios, C.A. (1999). *Recollections of Sexual Abuse: Treatment Principles and Guidelines*. New York: W.W. Norton.

Chu, J.A. (1998). *Rebuilding Shattered Lives*. New York: John Wiley & Sons.

Saakvitne, K.W, Gamble, S., Pearlman, L.A. & Lev, T.B. (2000). *Risking Connection: A Training Curriculum for Working with Survivors of Childhood Abuse*. Baltimore: The Sidran Press.

Herman, J. (1992). T*rauma and Recovery: The Aftermath of Violence — From Domestic Abuse to Political Terror*. New York: Basic Books.

Korn, D. L., & Leeds, A. M. (2002). Preliminary Evidence of Efficacy for emdr Resource Development and Installation in the Stabilization Phase of Treatment of Complex Posttraumatic Stress Disorder. *Journal of Clinical Psychology, 58(12)*, 1-23

Resources on Complex PTSR for Clients

Allen, J.G. (1995). *Coping with Trauma: A Guide to Self-Understanding*. Washington: American Psychiatric Press.

Rosenbloom, D., Williams, M.B. & Watkins, B.E. (1999). *Life After Trauma: A Workbook for Healing*. New York: Guilford.

Vermilyea, E.G. (2000). *Growing Beyond Survival: A Self-Help Toolkit for Managing Traumatic Stress*. Baltimore: The Sidran Press.

Williams, M.B. & Poijula, S. (2002). *The PTSD Workbook: Simple, Effective Techniques for Overcoming Traumatic Stress Symptoms*. Oakland, California: New Harbinger Publications.

Internet Resources

Sidran Institute
www.sidran.org

Sidran Institute is a non-profit organization that provides information to support people with traumatic stress conditions and to help educate mental health professionals and the public.

The PILOTS Database

www.ncptsd.org/publications/pilots/index.html

PILOTS is a bibliographical database covering Published International Literature on Traumatic Stress. A search function is available to locate the literature on PTSD and other mental-health sequelae of traumatic events.

International Society for Traumatic Studies

www.istss.org

The International Society for Traumatic Stress Studies offers fact sheets on traumatic loss and the emotional response both for professionals and for the public.

Glossary

Affect dysregulation: the inability to regulate feelings and emotional responses; significant difficulties dealing with emotions and impulses.

Affect regulation: the ability to experience, tolerate and integrate feelings.

Complex post-traumatic stress disorder (complex PTSD): consists of six dimensions of psychological functioning that are changed as a result of a person's developmental adaptations to a combination of ongoing sexual, physical or emotional abuse. These abuse experiences often take place in a context of neglect and chronic stress.

Conditioned emotional responses: An automatic response that a person has to a particular stimulus or similar stimuli (similar to the original abuse).

Constriction: a reduced range of expression and intensity of feelings.

Dissociation: a change in consciousness characterized by estrangement from the self or one's environment. Dissociation is also a defence mechanism to ward off the emotional impact of traumatic events and memories.

Dual awareness: the process of being able to be aware of one or more areas of experience simultaneously. This can be thought of as having one foot in the present, while the other foot is in the past.

Emotional lability: rapidly changing emotions.

Emotional valence: the weight or impact of emotions.

Empathic attunement: occurs when the therapist is attuned to the client's subjective experience (often sensing half-hidden meanings) and is able to communicate this understanding to the client.

Eye Movement Desensitization and Reprocessing (EMDR): a type of therapy that uses sets of eye movement or other forms of bilateral stimulation to try to help the client remember, neutralize, and resolve the upsetting memories at the root of current psychological disturbances. The use of EMDR has been adapted and expanded for other uses beyond trauma work, such as the development of inner strengths and resources, the treatment of addictions and eating disorders, and performance enhancement.

Fight-or-flight response: the activation of the sympathetic nervous system by a stressful event. When a person is trapped, he or she has a surge of physiological arousal — with no outlet for this arousal — resulting in agitation, tension and anxiety.

Fragmentation: feeling separated into different parts, or feeling the detachment of one or more parts of the self. People who fragment feel they are falling apart, losing their identity, etc.

Grounding: becoming firmly rooted in the present existence, or the "here and now."

Hyperarousal: being in a state of extreme psychological and physiological expectancy and readiness.

Hypermnesia: the opposite of amnesia; with hypermnesia, memories flood uncontrollably into a person's mind.

Hypervigilance: constant heightened awareness of one's surroundings to protect against potential harm or danger (i.e., feeling the need to be on guard all the time).

Hypoarousal: being unable to reach a state of psychological and physiological expectancy and readiness that is appropriate to a situation.

Mindfulness: the non-judgmental awareness and here-and-now observation of one's thoughts, emotions, sensations, and behaviours.

Normalizing: a reassuring reaction to disclosed traumatic experiences (or trauma responses) in a relaxed and matter-of-fact manner. This will decrease the likelihood that the client will feel singled out and stigmatized.

Post-traumatic stress disorder: see Complex post-traumatic stress disorder and Simple post-traumatic stress disorder.

Revictimization: multiple experiences of sexual violence, as well as the increased vulnerability to further sexual violence, most often resulting from an early experience of child sexual abuse.

Self-capacities: the inner abilities that allow a person to manage his or her inner world and maintain a coherent and cohesive sense of self.

Self-regulation: the ability to modulate or balance physiological arousal (i.e., to have all of one's emotional feelings within relatively comfortable limits).

Simple post-traumatic stress disorder (simple PTSD): post-traumatic stress resulting from a single traumatic event and not linked to any previous traumatic experiences (such as child sexual abuse, rape or a sudden loss).

Somatization: the development of persistent physical complaints that often defy medical explanation or intervention.

Therapeutic alliance: a relationship between the therapist and client, characterized by factors such as collaboration, containment, mutuality, etc.

Traumatic event: an extraordinary and overwhelming experience that is perceived as threatening to a person's life or physical integrity, and continues to exert negative effects on thinking (cognition), feelings (affects) and behaviour long after the event is in the past.

Traumatic response: a psychobiological reaction to a traumatic event, a traumatic response is characterized by discomfort and distress, and includes reactions such as hyperarousal, emotional numbing and re-experiencing responses. Not all traumatic events lead to trauma responses in all people.

Traumatic sexualization: the distorted shaping of a child's sexuality in developmentally inappropriate ways.

Trigger: any environmental or internal cue that serves as a reminder of a traumatic event — either directly or through a series of associations. A person who is triggered experiences the fight-or-flight response as if the event is happening in the present.

Vicarious trauma: the process by which mental health professionals have their own overwhelming responses to hearing about the terrible details of clients' abuse stories.

References

Abueg, F.R., Follette, V.M. & Ruzek, J.I. (Eds.). (1998). *Cognitive-Behavioural Therapies for Trauma*. New York: The Guilford Press.

Allen, J.G. (1995). *Coping with Trauma: A Guide to Self-Understanding*. Washington, DC: American Psychiatric Press.

American Psychiatric Association. (1994). *Diagnostic and Statistical Manual for Mental Disorders (4th ed.)* Washington, DC: Author.

Blaustein, M. E., Spinazzola, J., Simpson, W. & van der Kolk, B.A. (2000). *Psychological Sequelae of Early Trauma: Comorbid Diagnoses or Diagnostic Entity?* Paper presented at the 16th Annual Meeting of the International Society for Traumatic Stress Studies, San Antonio, TX.

Braun, B.G. (1988). The BASK Model of Dissociation. *Dissociation, 1*, 4–23.

Briere, J. (1992). *Child Abuse Trauma: Theory and Treatment of the Lasting Effects*. Newbury Park, CA: Sage Publications.

Briere, J. (1996). *Therapy for Adults Molested as Children: Beyond Survival*. (2nd ed.). New York: Springer Publishing.

Briere, J. (2002). Treating Adult Survivors of Severe Childhood Abuse and Neglect: Further Development of an Integrative Model. In J.E.B. Meyers, L. Berliner, J. Briere, T. Reid & C. Jenny (Eds.), *The APSAC Handbook on Child Maltreatment* (2nd ed.). Newbury Park, CA: Sage Publications.

Briere, J., Elliott, D.M., Harris, K. & Cotman, A. (1995). Trauma Symptom Inventory: Psychometrics and Association with Childhood and Adult Trauma in Clinical Samples. *Journal of Interpersonal Violence, 10*, 387–401.

Brothers, D. (1995). *Falling Backwards: An Exploration of Trust and Self Experience*. New York: W.W. Norton & Company, Inc.

Cardena, E. (1994). The Domain of Dissociation. In S.J. Lynn & J.W. Rhue (Eds.), *Dissociation: Clinical and Theoretical Perspectives* (pp. 15–31). New York: Guilford Press.

Carlson, E.A. (1998) A Prospective Longitudinal Study of Disorganized/Disoriented Attachment. *Child Development, 69*, 1107-1128.

Chu, J.A. (1998). *Rebuilding Shattered Lives*. New York: John Wiley & Sons.

Cohen, J.A., Perel, J.M., DeBellis, M.D., Friedman, M.J. & Putnam, F.W. (2002). *Treating Traumatized Children: Clinical Implications of the Psychobiology of Post-traumatic Stress Disorder.* Trauma, Violence & Abuse: A Review Journal, Vol. 3, No. 2. Thousand Oaks: Sage Publications.

Connors, R.E. (2000). *Self-Injury: Psychotherapy with People Who Engage in Self-Inflicted Violence.* North Vale, NJ: Jason Aronson.

Courtois, C.A. (1999). *Recollections of Sexual Abuse: Treatment Principles and Guidelines.* New York: W.W. Norton.

Davies, J.M. & Frawley, M.G. (1994). *Treating the Adult Survivors of Childhood Sexual Abuse.* New York: Basic Books.

Dolan, Y.M. (1991). *Resolving Sexual Abuse: Solution-Focused Therapy and Ericksonian Hypnosis for Adult Survivors.* New York: W.W. Norton.

Eichenbaum, H. & Cohen, N.J. (2001). *From Conditioning to Conscious Recollection: Memory Systems of the Brain.* Oxford, UK: Oxford University Press.

Elliott, D.M. (1994). Impaired Object Relations in Professional Women Molested as Children. *Psychotherapy, 31,* 79-86.

Felitti, V.J., Anda, R.F., Nordenberg, D., Williamson, D.F., Spitz, A.M., Edwards, V., Koss, M.P. & Marks, J.S. (1998). Relationship of Childhood Abuse and Household Dysfunction to Many of the Leading Causes of Death in Adults: The Adverse Childhood Experiences (ACE) Study. *American Journal of Preventive Medicine, 14,* 245-258.

Finkelhor, D. (1986). *A Sourcebook on Child Sexual Abuse.* Beverly Hills: Sage Publications.

Finkelhor, D. & Browne, A. (1985). The Traumatic Impact of Child Sexual Abuse: A Conceptualization. *American Journal of Orthopsychiatry, 55* (4), 530-541.

Friedman, M.J. (2000). *Post Traumatic Stress Disorder: The Latest Assessment and Treatment Strategies.* Kansas City: Compact Clinics.

Friedman, M.J., Lindy, J.D. & Wilson, J.P. (Eds.). (2001). *Treating Psychological Trauma & PTSD.* New York: The Guilford Press.

Gamble, S., Lev, B.T., Pearlman, L.A. & Saakvitne, K.W. (2000). *Risking Connection: A Training Curriculum for Working with Survivors of Childhood Abuse.* Lutterville, MD: The Sidran Press.

Gidycz, C.A., Hanson, K. & Layman, M.J. (1995). A Prospective Analysis of the Relationships among Sexual Assault Experiences. *Psychology of Women Quarterly, 19,* 5-29.

Harris, M. (1998). *Trauma, Recovery and Empowerment: A Clinician's Guide for Working with Women in Groups*. New York: The Free Press.

Haskell, L. (1997). *Revictimization in Women's Lives: An Empirical and Theoretical Account of the Links Between Child Sexual Abuse and Repeated Sexual Violence*. Unpublished doctoral dissertation, University of Toronto.

Haskell, L. (2001). *Bridging Responses: A Front-Line Worker's Guide to Supporting Women Who Have Post-Traumatic Stress*. Toronto: Centre for Addiction and Mental Health.

Hearst-Ikeda, D. (2000). CBT *Materials for Therapists and Clients. Cognitive Behavior Therapy for* PTSD *Stage II: Trauma Processing*. Boston: VA Boston Healthcare System.

Herman, J. (1992). *Trauma and Recovery: The Aftermath of Violence — From Domestic Abuse to Political Terror*. New York: Basic Books.

Kaschak, E. (1992). *Engendered lives: A New Psychology of Women's Experience*. New York: BasicBooks.

Leeds, A.M. (1997). In the Eye of the Beholder: Reflections on Shame, Dissociation, and Transference in Complex Posttraumatic Stress and Attachment Related Disorders. Principles of Case Formulation for EMDR Treatment Planning and the Use of Resource Installation. Paper presented at the EMDR International Association, San Francisco. Avalable: www.andrewleeds.net/presentations.html

Leeds, A.M. & Shapiro, F. (2000). EMDR and Resource Installation: Principles and Procedures for Enhancing Current Functioning and Resolving Traumatic Experiences. In Carlson, J. & Sperry, L. (Eds.), *Brief Therapy with Individuals and Couples*. Phoenix, AZ: Zeig, Tucker & Theisen, Inc.

Luxenberg, T., Spinazzola, J. & van der Kolk, B. A. (2001). Complex Trauma and Disorders of Extreme Stress (DESNOS) Diagnosis, Part I: Assessment. In *Directions in Psychiatry*. Long Island City, NY: The Hatherleigh Company, Ltd.

Luxenberg, T., Spinazzola, J., Hidalgo, J., Hunt, C. & van der Kolk, B.A. (2001). Complex Trauma and Disorders of Extreme Stress (DESNOS) Diagnosis, Part II: Treatment. In *Directions in Psychiatry*. Long Island City, NY: The Hatherleigh Company, Ltd.

Mandoki, C.A. & Burkhart, B.R. (1989). Sexual Victimization: Is There a Vicious Cycle? *Violence and Victims, 4* (3), 179–190.

Matsakis, A. (1994). *Post-Traumatic Stress Disorder: A Complete Treatment Guide*. Oakland, CA: New Harbinger Publications.

McCann, I.L. & Pearlman, L.A. (1990). *Psychological Trauma and the Adult Survivor: Theory, Therapy and Transformation.* New York: Brunner/Mazel.

McFarlane, A.C., van der Kolk, B.A. & Weisaeth, L. (Eds.). (1996). *Traumatic Stress: The Effects of Overwhelming Experience on Mind, Body and Society.* New York: The Guilford Press.

McLean, L. (2001). *The Relationship between Early Childhood Sexual Abuse and the Adult Diagnoses of Borderline Personality Disorder and Complex Posttraumatic Stress Disorder: Diagnostic Implications.* Paper presented at the Harvey Stancer Research Day, University of Toronto, Toronto, ON: Department of Psychiatry.

Meichenbaum, D. (1994). *A Clinical Handbook/Practical Therapist Manual for Assessing and Treating Adults with Post-Traumatic Stress Disorder.* Waterloo, ON: Institute Press.

Messler Davies, J. & Frawley, M.G. (1994). *Treating the Adult Survivor of Childhood Sexual Abuse: A Psychoanalytic Perspective.* New York: BasicBooks.

Messman, T.L & Long, P.J. (1996) Child Sexual Abuse and Its Relationship to Revictimization in Adult Women: A Review. *Clinical Psychology Review,* 16 (5), 397–420.

Miller, P.H. & Scholnick, E.K. (2000). *Toward a Feminist Developmental Psychology.* New York: Routledge.

Morrow, M. & Chappell, M. (1999). *Hearing Women's Voices: Mental Health Care for Women. Women's Health Reports.* Vancouver: British Columbia Centre of Excellence for Women's Health.

Nijenhuis, E.R.S. (1999). *Somatoform Dissociation: Phenomena, Measurement, and Theoretical Issues.* The Netherlands: Van Gorum & Co.

Ogden, P. & Minton, K. (2000). Sensorimotor Psychotherapy: One Method for Processing Traumatic Memory. *Traumatology,* VI (3), Article 3.

Pearlman, L.A. (2001). Treatment of Persons with Complex PTSD and Other Trauma-Related Disruptions of the Self. In J.P. Wilson, M.J. Friedman & J.D. Lindy (Eds.), *Treating Psychological Trauma and PTSD* (pp. 205–236). New York: Guilford Press.

Pearlman, L.A. & Saakvitne, K.W. (1995). *Trauma and the Therapist: Countertransference and Vicarious Traumatization in Psychotherapy with Incest Survivors.* New York: W.W. Norton.

Pelcovitz, D., van der Kolk, B.A. & Roth, S., et al. (1997). Development of a Criteria Set and a Structured Interview for Disorder of Extreme Stress (SIDES). *Journal of Traumatic Stress,* 10, 3–16.

Poijula, S. & Williams, M.B. (2002). *The PTSD Workbook: Simple, Effective Techniques for Overcoming Traumatic Stress Symptoms*. Oakland, CA: New Harbinger Publications.

Putman, F.W. (1989). *Diagnosis and Treatment of Multiple Personality Disorder*. New York: Guilford Press.

Ross, C.A.(1992). Childhood Sexual Abuse and Psychobiology. *Journal of Child Sexual Abuse, 1* (2).

Roth, S., Wayland, K. & Woolsey, M. (1990). Victimization History and Victim Assailant Relationship as Factors in Recovery from Sexual Assault. *Journal of Traumatic Stress, 3* (1), 169–180.

Rothschild, B. (2000). *The Body Remembers: The Psychophysiology of Trauma and Trauma Treatment*. New York: W.W. Norton.

Saakvitne, K.W., Gamble, S., Pearlman, L.A. & Lev, T.B. (2000). *Risking Connection: A Training Curriculum for Working with Survivors of Childhood Abuse*. Baltimore: Sidran Press.

Schore, A.N. (2001). The Effects of Early Relational Trauma on Right Brain Development, Affect Regulation, and Infant Mental Health. *Infant Journal of Mental Health,* 22, 201–269.

Siegel, D.J. (1999). *The Developing Mind*. New York: The Guilford Press.

Spinazzola, J., Blaustein, M., Kisiel, C. & van der Kolk, B. (2001). *Beyond PTSD: Further Evidence for a Complex Adaptational Response to Traumatic Life Events*. Paper presented at the American Psychiatric Association Annual Meeting, New Orleans.

Stanko, Elizabeth, A. (1990). *Everyday Violence: How Men and Women Experience Sexual and Physical Danger*. San Francisco: Harper/Collins.

Summit, R.C. (1983). The Child Sexual Abuse Accommodation Syndrome. *Child Abuse & Neglect,* 7, 177–193.

Ulman, R.B. & Brothers, D. (1988). *The Shattered Self: A Psychoanalytic Study of Trauma*. Hillsdale, NJ: The Analytic Press.

van der Kolk, B.A. (1989). The Compulsion to Repeat the Trauma: Re-enactment, Revictimization, and Masochism. *Psychiatric Clinics of North America,* 12 (2), 289–411.

van der Kolk, B.A., Perry, J.C. & Herman, J.L. (1991). Childhood Origins of Self-Destructive Behaviour. *American Journal Psychiatry,* 148, 1165–1671.

van der Kolk, B.A. (1994a). The Body Keeps the Score: Memory and the Evolving Psychobiology of Post-Traumatic Stress. *Harvard Review of Psychiatry, 1,* 253–65.

van der Kolk, B.A., & Fisler, R.E., (1994). Childhood Abuse & Neglect and Loss of Self-Regulation. *Bulletin of the Menninger Clinic, 58* (2).

van der Kolk, B.A., Roth, S. & Pelcovitz, D. (1994). Field Trials for DSM-IV, Post-Traumatic Stress Disorder II: Disorders of Extreme Stress. *American Journal of Psychiatry.*

van der Kolk, B.A. (1996). The Body Keeps the Score: Approaches to the Psychobiology of Posttraumatic Stress Disorder. In B.A. van der Kolk, A. McFarlane & L. Weisaeth (Eds.), *Traumatic Stress: The Effects of Overwhelming Experience on Mind, Body, and Society.* New York: Guilford Press.

van der Kolk, B. A. (2001). The Assessment and Treatment of Complex PTSD. In R. Yehuda (Ed.), *Traumatic Stress.* Washington, DC: American Psychiatric Press.

van der Kolk, B.A. (2002). Beyond the Talking Cure: Somatic Experience, Subcortical Imprints and the Treatment of Trauma. In F. Shapiro (Ed.), EMDR, *Promises for a Paradigm Shift.* New York, American Psychiatric Press.

Vermilyea, E.G. (2000). *Growing Beyond Survival: A Self-Help Toolkit for Managing Traumatic Stress.* Baltimore: The Sidran Press.

Weekes, C. (1984). *More Help for Your Nerves.* New York: Bantam.

Wilson, S., van der Kolk, B.A., Burbridge, J., Fisler, R. & Kradin, R. (1999). Phenotype of Blood Lymphocytes in PTSD Suggests Chronic Immune Activation. *Psychosomatics, 40,* 222–225.

Worell, J. & Remer, P. (1992). *Feminist Perspectives in Therapy: An Empowerment Model for Women.* Chichester, England: John Wiley & Sons.

Wyatt, G.E., Guthrie, D. & Notgrass, C.M. (1992). Differential Effects of Women's Child Sexual Abuse and Subsequent Sexual Revictimization. *Journal of Consulting and Clinical Psychology, 60* (2), 167–173.

Yehuda, R. (1998). Neuroendocrinology of Trauma and PTSD. *Psychological Trauma, 17.* American Psychiatric Press.

Young, J.E. (1999). *Cognitive Therapy for Personality Disorders: A Schema Focused Approach.* Practitioners Resource Series, 3rd Edition. New York: Professional Resource Exchange.